How *Yoga Works*, an introduction to somatic yoga, is a precious book, which acts as a bridge between both world hemispheres, East and West, by combining hatha and raja yoga, and elucidating the physical principles as well as the mental aspects of yoga practice.

The book can act as an inspiration for the layman as well as for the experienced yoga practitioner. A beautiful and comprehensive book, the language is so clear and noble in its simplicity that it enables even a layperson like myself to absorb it and to understand what it is about.

Almost every chapter in this wonderful book embraces a whole universe. Its general appeal is exemplified by the fact that it begins with a quote from an Indian guru, who stands on the summit—the top of the mountain—as well as a quote from a student, a beginner, who stands at its foot.

Yardena Alotin
Composer
Tel Aviv, Israel

How Yoga Works:

An Introduction to

Somatic

YOGA

How Yoga Works:

An Introduction to
Somatic
YOGA

Eleanor Criswell

FREEPERSON PRESS
NOVATO, CALIFORNIA

Dedicated to
Eleanor David and Norman Camp (my parents),
Peggy Granger, Thomas Hanna, and Miriam C. Bradley

Cover Design: CABA Design Office
Photos: Pamela Robertson
Interior Design & Typesetting: TBH/Typecast, Inc.
Printing & Binding: McNaughton & Gunn

Printed in the United States of America
First Edition: 1987

Published by
FREEPERSON PRESS
455 Ridge Road, Novato, CA 94947

Acknowledgments

Figures on pages 112, 118, 119, 120, 121, 123, 128, 132, 134, 135, 137, 138, 140, 142, 148, 150, 153, and 157 from *Survey of Functional Neuroanatomy* (second edition) by Bill Garoutte, PhD, MD. Copyright © 1987 by Jones Medical Publications. Reprinted by permission of the author and publisher.

Figures on pages 143 and 144 from *The Body of Life* by Thomas Hanna. Copyright © 1980 by Thomas Hanna. Publisher, Alfred Knopf. Reprinted by permission of the author.

Contents

Preface

Twenty-two years ago a book by Rammurti Mishra captured my imagination and the imagination of others. It was *The Fundamentals of Yoga*. In this book, Mishra wove together strands of medicine, psychology and raja yoga to show how yogic development related to the understandings of contemporary medicine and physiology. He also wrote a book which was entitled originally *A Textbook of Yoga Psychology*, retitled in paperback, *Yoga Sutras*. It was essentially Mishra's translation of Patanjali's *Yoga Sutras* (circa 400 B.C.), which is the classic treatise on raja or ashtanga yoga: yoga psychology. Other books on yoga are primarily about hatha yoga with scant attention paid to yoga psychology.

The excitement created by Mishra's book stemmed from the fact that he brought together many different areas of contemporary knowledge from the perspective of a medically educated, yogically trained Indian, and he showed us a glimpse of the wonders that are possible for the yogically trained person.

Since the publication of Mishra's book, there emerged a field of psychophysiology which included electrical physiological monitoring and change of physiological states through biofeedback training. These technological advances enabled yoga researchers to monitor the state of the yogi as well as observe the validity of their claim that the autonomic and other nervous systems have a capacity to learn. During the past 20 years, psychophysical research findings and yoga research per se have expanded rapidly. Yoga research has resulted in a strong substantiation of yoga's effectiveness and has supplied an impetus for yoga's widening acceptance as a part of contemporary life.

This is the tip of the iceberg of a legacy of information that has rapidly accrued during the past 20 years, scientific information that has increasingly enriched and transformed our conception of ourselves, of how our own bodies function, and how, finally, we can maintain our development and personally control our state of physical and mental health.

Psychologists, physicians, physical educators, physiologists — all, from their own perspectives, have been exploring a terrain that is rapidly becoming the same terrain: the human's capacity for self-regulation of psychophysical states.

What has become apparent is that there is a common view emerging that the human can understand and self-regulate the body far more easily than we dreamed possible. It is a view that is little short of revolutionary in terms of medicine, education, and psychotherapy—revolutionary in that it involves a turning away from the traditional view in the West of the separation of "mind" and "body" within the human. Within recent times, the weight of research evidence has tipped the balance on the scales toward a more integrated view of the human as self-regulating. It has fully validated the subjective view of the yoga practioner; indeed, it has catapulted yoga psychology fully into the present. Contemporary yoga psychology becomes then a somatic yoga. The word somatic refers to the living mind-body integration which is the hallmark of this approach to yoga psychology.

Put simply a new ball game has begun for yoga psychology and the psychophysiological sciences, both research and applied, that puts the human condition in a new, fascinating, and encouraging light. It is fascinating because it directly points to ourselves, and encouraging because the evidence says that humans, psychologically and physiologically, are capable of immensely more than we presently believe in regard to our capabilities for growth, self-regulation, intelligence, and self-healing. All of these are basic categories of yoga psychology and psychology in general, and they have now taken on new life.

This new conception of the nature of the human being centers in a unitary conception of the living being as a unified mind-body organism capable of self-regulated change and development.

The upshot is that we can, through an organized mind-body

training system, self-regulate ourselves toward maximum development, maintenance, and repair (or healing).

How Yoga Works is a catalogue and summary of this research and this emergent understanding. What constitutes a fully functioning human is a psychological question. It is also a philosophical, ethical, educational, and medical question. And it is a remarkable fact that our Western science, in opening up to a new perspective on human life, has also begun to join hands with ancient human understandings that are primitive, that are Eastern, that are religious and mystical.

How Yoga Works is a book that brings yoga research out of the laboratories into the lives of individual humans, giving them a positive, hopeful, and intimate understanding of who they are as mortal beings who share the common experience of being self-conscious exemplars of an ancient and common developmental task and path. Yoga psychology is infinitely more understandable than it has been ever before. So many sciences are converging toward a common understanding of ourselves that a description of this convergence can now be made that is within the grasp of the average person.

This book will enable you to develop a basic understanding of yoga psychology or somatic yoga. It will explore entering the path, the goals or outcomes of yoga, the ethical principles of yoga, the basic postures, breathing exercises, progressive relaxation, concentration, meditation, Samadhi or the state of union, the physiology of somatic yoga, how the asanas work, the senses and concentration training, altered states of consciousness and the kundalini exprience, yoga and parapsychology, and somatic yoga as a way of life. The appendix includes a suggested somatic yoga training program. The main emphasis is on developing your personal yoga.

How Yoga Works is designed to be a treasure trove of information, self-understanding, training experiences and positive hope about the possibilities available for training the fully functioning, integrated mind-body person—you.

I would like to thank the yogis who have so generously contributed to my development and understanding of yoga: Dr. Rammurti Mishra, Swami Muktanada, Swami Vishnudevananda, and many others with whom I have had contact over the years. Some have visited our campus and guest-taught my Psychology of Yoga class; some spoke on campus such as Swami Satchitananda, Ram Das, and others. Dr. Haridas Chaudhuri was a valuable bridge between East and West and offered strong encouragement to me in making that bridge. I would also like to thank the hundreds of Sonoma State University students, faculty, and staff who have attended my Psychology of Yoga class over the past 20 years. All are my teachers.

For any endeavor that requires a sustained effort over time, such as writing a book (this one took approximately 16 years to complete), a caring support system is essential. I would like to thank my dear family, friends, and colleagues—Jane Bowerman, Norman M. Camp, Francis Criswell, Hazel Criswell, June Criswell, Victor Daniels, Thomas David, Sydney Fleischer, Richard Ajathan Gero, Don Hamachek, Tad Hanna, T. George Harris, Allegra Hiner, Samuel Hiner, Antoinette Jourard, Sidney Jourard, Marsha Joyce, Michael Joyce, Charles Merrill, Susan O'Grady, Logan Patterson, Mildred Patterson, Charles Posey, Kendall Posey, Neil Russack, Stephen Wall, Joan Wolf and many others for their caring, interest, and encouragement.

I would like to thank my friend Thomas Hanna for his continual support and encouragement and editorial comments. I would also like to thank Marsha Calhoun for her editorial suggestions. The photographs by Pamela Robertson are deeply appreciated. I am also grateful to Jay Daniel for the use of his studio and his assistance. Bill Garoutte's contributions to the functional neuronatomical material are invaluable. I am grateful to Bill Turner and the others at Typecast for beautifully guiding, typesetting, and formatting the book. I want to thank Christine Dunham and Craig Bergquist for their thoughtful cover design.

PART ONE

Entering the Path

1

Entering the Path

Enter the Path! There spring the healing streams
    Quenching all thirst! there bloom th' immortal flowers
Carpeting all the way with joy! there throng
    Swiftest and sweet hours.

Edwin Arnold

Yoga has opened my eyes to the void of the part of my mind which has been clouded with cobwebs all of my life. It will continue to keep me more young, healthy, and alive. It has helped and will help me gain self-confidence that I never previously imagined. It has and will continue to help me find myself along the everlasting pathway of my existence. I am the creator of the universe and I must learn to create beautiful things.

Yoga student

Yoga is a Sanscrit word, *yug*. Yug means yoke or union. It means, in essence, the unification or re-unification of the self with the universal Self. (This unification seems necessary because we perceive ourselves to be separate.) It also means the re-unification of the person—mentally, physically, and emotionally. In its ultimate sense, it refers to the reunification of humankind with the universe or cosmic consciousness or the Absolute. It is the discipline and training of the human's embodied being so that it evolves toward what it is capable of becoming. Yoga seeks to provide physical and mental training experiences to further refine the soma (unified mind-body). There are many approaches to yoga.

Selecting Your Yoga (the "way" that suits you)

How do you select your yoga? Because there are many yogas, there is a yoga for everyone who practices it. Why? Easterner,

Westerner, or cross-cultural, no two people can duplicate the yogic orientation exactly. Yoga—classic, contemporary, eclectic—comes in many forms. Some students work with a guru; some students, alone. There being many ways, it is important to find the way that most reflects your inner being.

Among the approaches to yoga are hatha, raja, jnana, karma, and bhakti. Hatha yoga is the way of physical discipline. Raja yoga is the approach which uses mental discipline. Jnana yoga emphasizes knowledge as the yogic way. Karma yoga specializes in action in the world—selfless service. Bhakti is considered the way of love and devotion. All are attempts to leave the alienated state of existence and regain the sense of union with the ground of Being (Atman rejoined with Brahman).

Chaudhuri (1975, p. 236) lists the following yoga disciplines which evolved from the fifth century B.C. to the 18th century A.D.: The yoga of breath control (hatha); the yoga of mind control (raja); the yoga of action (karma); the yoga of love (bhakti); the yoga of knowledge (jnana); the yoga of "being-energy" (kundalini); the yoga of integral consciouness (pura). He says that "the ultimate goal of all of the above self-disciplines is blissful union with the Self in its transcendental dimension of oneness with timeless Being." They are different in their approach, but they are all moving toward the practice of self-realization and ego-transcendence. Chaudhuri's conception of "integral yoga" stressed the necessity of moving beyond development of the self to the use of that self in the development of society.

Integral yoga bridges the gap between transcendence and participation in the world. Chaudhuri describes samadhi as "the experience of freedom, immortality, transcendence of subject-object dichotomy, inexpressible bliss, limitless expansion of consciousness" (1975, p. 246). Immediately following self-realization, there is a brief period of inaction followed by a new kind of action. This action, empowered by Being-energy, is used along the lines of your perceived destiny. Chaudhuri says that "the unmistakable mark of this authentic self-realization [the individual's] would be his egoless dedication to cosmic welfare" (p. 252).

What is Somatic Yoga?

The yoga presented in this book is called somatic because it aims toward mind-body unification. It uses hatha yoga practices coupled with raja yoga practices. It includes the principles of psychophysiology, awareness techniques, visualization exercises, etc. It also draws heavily from the biofeedback research literature for actual effects of the practices. It is a composite yoga which aims toward increased unification of your mind and body during all of the experiences in daily life. A yoga for modern times, it is designed to be blended with your daily activities and lifestyle.

Somatic yoga has to do with the evolution of the person— mind, body, and spirit. It leans heavily on sensing your life's work or destiny. The various practices facilitate being able to hear more and more messages from your inner wisdom or guidance.

Your Yoga Teacher

It is really great to have a yoga teacher. When I began my yoga practice with meditation, I lived in Kentucky. That was many years ago. I had only books and my inner responses to tell me when I was hot or cold vis-a-vis "The Path." What I used at that time was my inner teacher. As Ram Das points out in his book *Be Here Now*, it is not essential to have a teacher physically present. Your guru can be present, distant, or no longer living on this plane of existence. You do not even need to know who he or she is or whether you have one or not. He or she will still be assisting you. If you feel drawn to various teachers, present or past, chances are they are assisting you, directly or indirectly.

When you are ready, the saying goes, your guru or teacher will appear. It is not necessary to traverse the world; your teacher will come to you. In fact, it is more likely to happen if you remain centered in your practice rather than seeking far and wide. It will happen, when you are ready. A guru or teacher will visit your area or you may visit his. If you feel suitably drawn to him—he seems genuinely to communicate to you, the deepest you—then perhaps you may wish to be initiated by him. In the initiation ceremony, he may give you a personal mantra (sacred syllable) or other specialized practices. This is not an absolute necessity for yogic development. It does seem to facilitate one's practice and development, however. There seems to be a special effect which occurs when you surrender to a divine presence. Even so, you should still retain your common sense under all circumstances. Evaluate the directions of your teacher with discretion.

As a college professor, I feel the need to offer practices from many yogic orientations. The right guru for me would respect and include all these aspects in his teachings.

Michael Murphy, co-founder of the Esalen Institute and a mystic athlete, feels that the contemporary sadhana (liberating discipline) is eclectic, including aspects from many orientations. The opposite view is held by some gurus. They feel that searching too widely is like trying to dig a well by starting over and over in different places, never getting anywhere in depth.

You can use books as teachers, friends as teachers; even your local yoga teacher can serve as your guru. The important thing is to be open, to listen to your inner responses, and to incorporate those practices which seem productive. Those practices that prove themselves to you can become part of your way of life.

In conclusion, I do not think we need to, nor can we, become Indian yogis—the cultural diffusion and translation cannot be complete. Here on our side of the blood-brain barrier of cultural differences, we can evolve our own yoga, one more suited to our bodies, our needs, and our culture.

The Effect of the Right Guru Upon a Chela (student)

"The guru is one who has experienced divine freedom in his consciousness, and knows the meaning by which it can be attained" (Wood, 1962, p. 12). At best, the guru is a highly evolved being. He, sometimes she, has attained some level of enlightenment and can by that grace show you some of the approaches you can use to begin or continue your own development. The guru will set an example; you will follow to the degree that you are able. I find this kind of process very effective for some people. Beginners, people at certain stages of their development, and those with dependent personalities seem to gravitate to the guru. Although you can learn yoga best with a guru or teacher, in the final analysis you are your own teacher. As you listen to the teachings and your body's responses to them, you will incorporate your own interpretations into your lifestyle.

When you are in the presence of a teacher suited to you, you will feel a special response within yourself. This has been called the quickening of the spirit. It manifests itself in soft, subtle vibrations within your body, gently heightened temperature, and mood elevation. In short, you experience an altered state of consciousness. Before I experienced this in the presence of a guru, I had only an intellectual understanding of how this could be so. During this encounter with your guru, there is, supposedly, a prana (energy) exchange. You either resonate empathically or actually receive/perceive the energy. If such an energy exchange actually does occur, it is not by any means that we can now measure technologically. Let us keep an open mind as our scientists explore subtler and subtler forms of energy. Perhaps they will someday validate this subjective experience.

> A mature spiritual guide (guru) sees to it that the disciple does not become emotionally fixated upon him. His main job is to help the disciple to discover the divine guru within the disciple's own unconscious psyche. As soon as the disciple learns to stand on his own feet, capable of treading the right path leading to the ultimate goal, the guru gracefully parts company, liberating the disciple from his last emotional bonds. . . . The powerful (siddha) guru can give something which nobody else indeed can give, not even a scholar or a philosopher or a psychiatrist. He can communicate or transmit the power of transcendental love which awakens the latent psychonuclear energy, or ignites the dormant spiritual spark in the disciple (Chaudhuri, 1975, p. 254).

When it is awakened, it feels something like a high-voltage electric charge. It facilitates spiritual awakening. Freeing the disciple is the next step. Guru-dependent self-realization is not the answer. Some individuals may be totally unsuited to independent living, however. Your own true Self is your ultimate guru.

Chaudhuri (1975) feels that consciousness is the outgrowth of an evolution of the human nervous system. As the human continues to evolve he becomes capable of the leap toward an understanding of Being: at that point he experiences the state of oneness with Being. Chaudhuri lists the following varieties of mystic experience of yogis: (1) the experience of the Self as transempirical (beyond experience) subject; (2) the experience of the Self as pure transcendence beyond subject-object; (3) the experience of the creative ground of all existence; (4) the experience of the oneness of all existence; (5) the experience of the eternal Thou; and (6) the experience of the transpersonal Being-energy.

Yoga is used by various people for various purposes. Some people are interested in spiritual development. Their interest is primarily in yoga for spiritual culture. Others are interested in it for its effect on the physical self. They may be considered physical culturists. Either orientation is legitimate if it fits the needs of the person's basic psychological type. Yoga is like a cafeteria. You should take what suits you. Do not be disturbed by what does not. I have frequently stated as I presented the topic of the kriya yoga cleansing practices to my classes that I did not think I would ever find them the next most logical thing in my development. Recently, I heard a student of mine recount the wonders of these practices, reporting how breathing and meditation were facilitated. These kriya yoga practices were taught by an exceptional guru then in residence in California. I began to feel my attitude toward kriya yoga opening. I could almost sense that at some point even these practices might become part of my sadhana.

To find the yoga that suits you, follow this rule: listen carefully to yourself and what you feel drawn toward. Because we frequently overlook our inner direction in the din of external commands, we must practice listening repeatedly. To begin an approach, to learn its basic principles, to evolve away from it—all are a part of the process of finding your personal yoga. Sometimes, as you follow your unique path, you return to a method you explored earlier in your development. From your exploration comes a deeper understanding of your earlier practices. When you unify your practices, they will come together in your personal approach.

Yoga is a path, a way, a lifestyle. Through yoga you can normalize the functions of your entire organism. Body, mind, and emotions are brought into harmony and balance. There is a return to homeostasis. Yogic practices—physical movements, mental exercises, breathing patterns—provide an ongoing level of equilibrium or momentary rebalancing measures. Yoga is for life.

The key to yoga is practice; those who practice yoga achieve results. It is not limited to the talented few, but to those who sincerely devote a portion of each day to practice. Regardless of your goals for beginning yoga, you will be led into a fuller realization of many of your capacities if you practice faithfully.

Yoga can be viewed in another way: as an alchemical process. Not only is yoga a modification of behavior, it is also a recombination of your body's chemicals. With the recombination of body chemicals, the transmutation of your "base" self into your finer/higher self occurs.

Yoga is a personal alchemical process. Alchemy is the ancient practice of combining chemicals in an attempt to create gold out of baser metals which was the forerunner of modern chemistry, and which was perhaps also designed to evolve the consciousness of the alchemist. Through yoga, you can transform your self. The practices are like recipes: a pinch of this and a dash of that. The biochemical changes which accompany muscular effort, changes in the oxygen and carbon dioxide balance through special breathing patterns, the amount of time spent in each posture (cumulative effect), the effect of the difference of the flow of gravity—all contribute to the crucible of your evolving self. The chemical combination of your diet also contributes; environmental suggestions determine how that nutrition is used by your body. Gradually, you are transformed into your healthiest and most divine self.

Yoga Journal

It is a good idea to keep a yoga journal. In your yoga journal, you will want to keep a record of some of the insights, experiences, and ideas which come to you. Dreams are another source of inspiration and development; you will want to capture some of these. The verbal aspect present in writing is not meant to distract you from the experience itself, it merely helps make more conscious the significant aspects of your development. It is a way of learning more about yourself as your unconscious speaks to you through your written communication.

As you begin to keep your yoga journal, you will learn more about the way you want to go about it. In other words, the experience will guide you; the process will unfold. You will begin to remember more of your dreams. You will have more flashes of insight. It is as if some aspect of your self knew that it was appreciated. That its wisdom is being acted upon. Therefore, thoughts come more frequently to you. Keeping a journal "primes the pump," as it were, facilitates the flow, frees the creative forces within you.

Your yoga journal serves as a unifying collection of your thoughts on yoga. These reflections cry to be shared with someone—even if it is only your self to your self. Especially, if it is your self to your self. Some people prefer to keep yoga a nonverbal experience. If that is the case with you, you may prefer to keep your journal in an artistic or poetic form. Whatever form you choose, your yoga journal will serve as feedback to you of the effects of your practice. It also serves as a meditative experience when approached in that fashion. It will give you a sense of your progress along the yogic path.

2

The Goals or Outcomes of Yoga

Success in yoga comes quickly to those who are intensely energetic.

Patanjali

My aim in daily yoga is about an hour a day; usually I follow the same warm-ups and postures we do in class as a whole. My personal yoga is more centered on using yoga in interpersonal situations where I find it has greatly helped me; that is, in situations where I feel uncomfortable, nervous or even frightened.

Yoga student

We will now explore the goals of yoga practice from the perspective of contemporary psychological research. I will expand on each one so that you can see some of the reality behind the goal or claim. Yogis I have known do not necessarily exemplify these aspects. Each yogi is a human being; each has his unique character structure. The ultimate goal of yoga is union with the All. Ernest Wood, in his book, *Yoga*, feels that most aspirants to the yogic way are inclined to postpone the ultimate goal. Knowing that the light of it illumines the way, they content themselves with lesser goals. The lesser goals of the practice of yoga include: peace of mind and heart; power of will, love, and intellect; direct influence of the mind upon the body and the world outside the body; psychic abilities of various kinds; control of mind and power of concentration; control of emotions (removal of worry, pride, anger, fear, lust, and greed); bodily health, suppleness, beauty, and longevity; and the prevention and removal of psychosomatic dangers and troubles (Wood, 1959, p. 36).

Whereas the ultimate goal of yoga is union with cosmic consciousness, ultimate reality, the Absolute, etc., these intermediary goals or gains are possible:

1. *Peace of mind.* Through meditation practices and the gradual balancing of physiological systems, you become able to put to rest some of the agitations and preoccupations of your mind. With relaxation frequently comes a shift toward parasympathetic nervous system dominance. The parasympathetic nervous system is associated with the activities of the brain's anterior hypothalamus and the milder emotions.

Years ago, I remember driving down the street with my family. I was leaning over from the backseat to the front. I was about fourteen at the time. I asked my mother to guess what I wanted most. She was surprised, and I think saddened, to find that at fourteen what I wanted most was peace of mind. I don't know whether "peace of mind" is something you want. Many people I know would gladly do whatever it took to achieve it. Yoga is a tremendous comfort and aid to achieving internal peace. To be of help to others you must begin with yourself.

2. *Will and motivation.* There are a number of theories of motivation. The theory which seems to have most relevance to our exploration of yoga has to do with the activation/arousal of the organism by your reticular activating system.

As Butter says (1968, p. 138),

> Whenever homeostatic regulation involves overt behavior, we speak of that behavior as being motivated. The concept of motivation, then, refers to behavioral adjustments which satisfy needs of the body. Corresponding to many internal needs there is assumed to be a particular motive or drive. . . . A drive is customarily thought of as an internal state arising from a need and provoking consummatory responses, such as eating or drinking (mediated by hypothalamic mechanisms that regulate internal states).

One of the things that you may notice, during sustained yoga practice, is the increased capacity to set goals and then move toward achieving them.

3. *Love*. One of the things you may notice as you practice yoga is an increased capacity to love. You may notice this with regard to special persons in your life or toward people in general. You may even feel an increased love toward your environment and even objects in your environment. You may feel an increased love of life. You may notice an increased capacity to love yourself.

One of the reasons that you may experience an increase in loving feelings has to do with the shift toward the parasympathetic nervous system dominance which is characteristic of the pleasant emotions. You will also experience a sense of decreased ego boundaries and the feeling of merging with persons or objects. With this blending comes a feeling of kinship and the beauty inherent in the person or object. There is often a feeling of gratitude.

4. *Increased intelligence*. Intelligence is difficult to define. It is essentially your ability to function effectively in society. To increase effective intelligence, it is necessary to keep your mind active. Through yoga it is possible to provide physiological experiences which increase circulation to the brain. It encourages good nutrition for the brain. It is possible through concentration exercises we mentioned to increase the effective use of your mental capacity. That we only use a small percentage of our mental capacity is an oft-repeated truism.

5. *Psychic faculties*. For a long time practitioners of yoga have reported psychic experiences. The experiences that they report run the gamut from telepathic to psychokinetic experiences. You probably will not experience dramatic changes in your psychic abilities, but you may experience those at the lower end of the continuum, such as increased empathic responses to other people, increased feelings of understanding what other people are thinking, or the increased feeling for the flow of events before they happen.

6. *Concentration*. In our culture and in our educational systems we do very little to teach concentration or attention. Many individuals spontaneously learn and others are taught bits and pieces of how to concentrate. It is a valuable experience to learn how to focus

one's mind and concentrate. Yoga practice helps develop concentration skills both physiologically and psychologically.

7. *Control of emotions.* Many people are trying to learn how to experience their emotions more intensely and more authentically. There are, however, situations in which it is very valuable to control your emotions. To reduce irritation and anger, to maintain peace of mind, to spend more of your time in a generalized happy state facilitates your health and the health and happiness of others. Yoga, because of its capacity to shift into the parasympathetic nervous system state, is an aid toward control of emotions.

8. *Bodily health, suppleness, beauty, and longevity.* Through yoga practice you may notice changes in your general state of health. You will probably notice this in the decrease in the number of incidences of illness during any given period of time. Correspondingly, if you leave off your yoga practice for a while, you will quite possibly notice an increase in illness. An increase in suppleness (flexibility) is very noticeable when you are engaging in sustained yoga practice. When you first begin to do yoga, you will notice considerable stiffness and soreness during and after practice. As you become more adept at doing the postures you will notice your suppleness increasing. This increased flexibility will be noticeable while you are doing your postures and during the day with other movements. If you stop doing your postures regularly for a while, you will notice a return of stiffness. When you begin to do your postures again, you will notice that you quickly return to your original suppleness.

When you are practicing your yoga regularly, you will notice an increase in your own natural beauty. Observable skin tone changes will occur. Skin blemishes will gradually decrease. You will have a glow of health that others will remark upon. In addition, the texture of your hair and nails will seem to improve. A weight normalization will occur. Individuals who are overweight will lose weight; individuals who are underweight will gain weight. Your facial expressions will become lovelier as you are happier and more at peace with yourself.

Longevity as the result of yoga is something that I have yet to see demonstrated. It is said that advanced yogis do gain longevity, but that they then choose the times of their deaths, when they choose to go into samadhi. What we can observe is that the yoga practitioner will probably live out his life with greater health and mobility in the world. Yoga practice is said to retard the effects of aging. With this we can see why long-time yoga practitioners behave with more youthful vigor.

9. *The prevention and removal of psychosomatic dangers and troubles.* Psychosomatic diseases are those physical problems that seem to have a psychological component. It seems that the result of your behavior or psychological state has an impact over time on your physiological state. Psychosomatic complaints have been said to include asthma, various kinds of headaches, gastrointestinal difficulties, hypertension, and others. Many of these complaints are the result of the body's reaction to stress over a long period of time. Yoga practice enables you to shift toward a parasympathetic nervous system dominance, the maintenance and repair system, and homeostasis. This shift is from the stress state to one of relaxation. With a more easy return to homeostasis following stress, you are less likely to stay in a prolonged stress state leading to psychosomatic complaints. Therefore, yoga practice will enable you to maintain a state of bodily health which tends to prevent psychosomatic difficulties. Also, with training in achieving homeostasis there is a reduction of the factors contributing to existing psychosomatic complaints.

Contraindications for Yoga Practice

Contraindications for yoga practice concern the circumstances under which yoga would not be beneficial. For those persons who are psychotic or borderline, it may encourage hallucinatory experiences by lowering physiological defenses which they have developed.

Yoga can lead some individuals to dissociative experiences. It is valuable under certain circumstances to be able to dissociate, but it is equally valuable to be able to be alert and connected to your experiences. Persons who have a tendency to withdraw may be encouraged in that direction by intense periods of meditation. Chaudhuri (1975) lists the following dangers on the path of yoga: (1) the danger of extreme introversion; (2) the danger of spiritual hedonism or gluttony; (3) the danger of regression; (4) the danger of emotional fixation on the guru; and (5) the danger of self-mutilation.

Having discussed the indications and contraindications for yoga practice, you are fully informed as to what you might expect. With this in mind, you can decide if yoga would be appropriate for you or someone with whom you are working. It is important to know the benefits of yoga, not so that you will be too goal-conscious, but so that you can allow those developments to flower through enhanced awareness of them.

gized, unified, this may have positive or negative effects, depending on your goals.

There are two ways of approaching yamas and niyamas: to decide to follow them or to evolve toward them. Although well intentioned, the first approach is practically guaranteed to fail. But why? When you have decided to follow them, when they are a departure from your ordinary behavior, when you have had very little experience with them, it is difficult to remember the rules consistently. The New Year's resolution is well-intended; its period of resolve, shortlived. Few can form a reasonable New Year's resolution, fewer still can maintain it.

What's the second approach? The second approach is more natural. You can change briefly psychologically, but not physiologically. Your muscle tone and your endocrine balance, your brain waves and focus of attention can be changed through physical practices. When your physiology—the yogic body—is altered, your behavior will be altered. When you are relaxed, focused, and content, you do not need to remember your intentions vigilantly. You need only to behave as naturally as possible, according to your true desires. You might keep the yamas and niyamas in mind, but you need not make a conscious effort to observe them.

First let's look at the yamas or abstentions. The yamas include: (a) non-injury, (b) truthfulness, (c) non-theft, (d) spiritual conduct, and (e) non-greed. What do they mean? What they mean can best be understood with the aid of several concepts. The first concept is the law of karma. Karma refers to the law of cause and effect. Just as the actions you engage in radiate out from you, so too will they return to affect you at some later time. The second concept has to do with how the particular action will affect your state of consciousness or psychophysiological state at the time.

Non-injury

The first yama refers to the non-injury of any living creature in thought, word, or action. Diet and lifestyle, personal and interpersonal interactions, work and play are areas in which non-

3

Yamas: Things to Avoid

Satisfactory spiritual growth is not possible without a harmonious and peaceful environment. Social position, physical strength, and mental brilliance are of no avail for lasting happiness, if there is constant discord and friction with those who belong to our social orbit. Ethico-religious ideas, even when they are imperfectly and inadequately formulated, have at least a limited value insofar as they emphasize man's organic relationship to society. According to Patanjali, there are ten fundamental ethico-religious principles which may be described as the imperatives of the authentic self.

Haridas Chaudhuri

It's funny that yoga, a very private and inward practice, should help me so much to open up and accept other people.

When I come to class, I am in my city mode, going fast, not too personal, kind of guarded. Without fail, during and after yoga class I feel so much more camaraderie with the people around me.

With the physical benefits of relaxation *and* alertness, I feel this attitude is the most enduring and important aspect of my daily living. Through the entire semester, this opening up and reaching out towards others has been a real key to new doors.

Yoga student

When you begin to learn yoga, it is important to touch bases with yamas and niyamas. The yamas—abstentions—are concerned with behaviors to avoid. Not only do you avoid the behavior, but also related thoughts. The niyamas are observances—things to do, ten rules to follow. Why rules? As you develop toward increased concentration, you develop toward greater efficiency in your actions. As you are more focused, ener-

injury is to be practiced. A diet which precludes eating anything that does not fall from the plant of its own accord is an extreme example.

However vivid or dramatic or extreme the practice, this prohibition has mainly to do with karma. Positive or negative, karma refers to the action which finally returns to impact on you. Physiologically and psychologically, the effect of engaging in an injurious act is on yourself in a sympathetic nervous system dominant state. The sympathetic nervous system state includes biochemical changes (adrenalin and noradrenalin), electrochemical changes, muscle tone changes, and others. The systemic effects last several hours after the original stimulus. For these reasons, the personal price of injury to others is frequently considered not worth it.

Truthfulness

As with the other rules, this one has karmic and physiological implications. A boomerang effect, the law of karma indicates that your acts return to haunt you. Your untruthfulness will lead to untruthfulness toward you. You will not know if you can trust others. You know you are untrustworthy; others, therefore, will be equally untrustworthy.

What is the physiological effect of non-truthfulness? Two factors operate in the body's response to non-truthfulness. The first, most immediate effect concerns the physiological reaction that most people have when they are lying. That is the origin of the use of the lie detector or polygraph. Sensitive and responsive, the polygraph, in this case, is used to measure changes in the galvanic skin response. These changes reflect arousal or excitation. Changes in arousal are accompanied by increases in sympathetic nervous system activity. This change in sympathetic nervous system activity also accompanies the orienting reflex—the reflex response to novel stimuli. Most people react psychophysiologically to lying; some do not.

Once you have told a lie you must then remember it. Sometimes you have to tell several lies. The additional lies are designed to insure consistency. Then you have to remain vigilant. You must be able to remember the fabricated reality at any time in the future. As you engage in sustained yoga practice, you will notice yourself staying closer to your true version of reality.

The central nervous system requires new stimulation. The organism is always seeking novel stimulation. It is alert to any change in the environmental stimulation. This alertness takes the form of what seems like a matching system. The matching system compares the internal model of reality with the outside reality; it alerts the organism when there is a discrepancy. The organism is shifted by the orienting reflex (a brief sympathetic nervous system activation) toward greater arousal, greater alertness. These effects last for several hours afterwards. A lie is a definite mismatch between the real situation and the fabricated one. This artificial mismatch causes an alerting of the organism. The person who lies knows the true information and deliberately substitutes false information.

Yoga is an attempt to become increasingly calm and relaxed; this is a shift toward parasympathetic nervous system dominance. To the yogi, untruth in thought, word or deed which creates a sympathetic nervous system discharge is more trouble than it is worth.

Non-theft

Theft refers to taking what does not belong to you. This means stealing in thought, words or deeds. It can be seen either karmically or physiologically in the toll it takes on the person who engages in it. For a variety of reasons, the yogi practices non-theft.

On the karmic level, taking what does not belong to you means that sooner or later you will receive the same treatment. It means that you live in a world of thieves because that is the kind of attitude you will project on others. It is the only way you know a human to be. You will always have to be on your guard against others stealing your goods. This means that you are in a high state of stress all the time because of your need for vigilance.

On a physiological level, the thief goes through a variety of physiological changes during the act of stealing. Then there is the concern for hiding the stolen goods and avoiding being caught. There is the awareness that what is possessed does not belong as part of his life, did not come to him by natural means, may not even suit his lifestyle. There is the lack of comfort with the alien object. All of this leads to a state of sympathetic nervous system dominance of varying degrees whenever he deals with the object. For the yogi, this is excess baggage. It takes him away from his desired state of easy, relaxed living and harmony with his environment. It also reinforces the effects of other yamas and niyamas such as greed.

Spiritual Conduct

Although it sounds positive, this yama actually refers to a negative state: sexual abstinence. Contemporary students of yoga need to be wary of the culture-bound origins of yoga's antisexual stance.

Put in its most radical form, spiritual conduct is a prescription that presumably enhances asceticism by the conservation of sexual energy. This yama is designed to turn one away from squandering sexual energies that should, instead, be devoted to the attainment of a higher consciousness. The tradition has it that by converting sexual energies into spiritual energies there is a resultant increase in kundalini and an enhancement of consciousness.

This tradition of sexual abstinence was, of course, bound up with the Hindu tradition of four life stages and the fact that the transition is from the stage of householder to that of the sadhu who has given up the role of householder. The role of husband, father and provider ended all at the same time – the sexual role was abandoned along with the forsaking of wife and occupation. It was the beginning of man's final stage of life: the trek toward nirvana and death. And nothing should stand in the way of this noble aspiration.

But for anyone outside of the traditional restraints of Indian culture, this yama makes little sense. Must one abandon mate, children, home and occupation in order to proceed on the yogic path? Certainly not. The yama of spiritual conduct presumes that an orderly discipline has been chosen for one's life, and this can be accomplished by balancing one's inner development against one's inter-personal relationships and one's professional life. In our own culture, it would be best to think of this yama as anti-promiscuity.

And for the notion that the saving of sexual energies transfers these energies to a higher consciousness: there is no basis for it. Abstinence does not "save" energy, but depletes and weakens it. This would make for a consciousness that was not so much higher as it was less vital. But there has been a great deal of debate on this issue with some maintaining that sexual abstinence creates greater intensity to the yogic life and others maintaining the opposite.

Once we remove this issue from the context of Indian culture, it seems a moot point. The dispute is likely a difference in personal preference and will always remain such.

But for most non-Indians choosing to practice yoga the issue of sexual abstinence is no issue at all. One can sincerely pursue the yogic path with a purely positive attitude about one's physiological needs. Somatic yoga sees sexual expression as an integral part of a healthy, balanced lifestyle.

Non-Greed

Non-greed refers to being able to meet and deal with events as they present themselves. It is a state of being non-attached, free from covetousness and possessiveness.

All material objects are transitory. To be passionately attached to material objects means to be attached to the transitory. Material objects are distractions from the main purpose of life. Although they are tantalizing, attachment to them can only cause grief as each passes away.

Have you experienced greed? Desiring more and more, you

cannot satify your desire. As you acquire the desired possessions, you find the joy is gone. Then the passion is for the next acquisition. Upon possessing it, the fulfillment you thought the possession would bring is absent.

With the experience of greed comes sympathetic nervous system arousal. You are mobilized toward acquisition and stimulus change; you are not able to achieve peace of mind. The more you hoped to find peace of mind in the flux of life, the less you are able to find it as you focus on acquisition. The King Midas touch— everything you touch turns to gold—seems to be your lot. Everything you acquire/touch ceases to have life for you—as you acquire it, it begins to degenerate.

As you become nonattached to material possessions, you can then have as much as you need for the conduct of your life. It is a paradox. When you are needy, you cannot have what you need. When you no longer need it, you get it. The movement toward nonattachment is rewarded, the movement toward attachment is not. Painful or repetitious, it is all part of life's learning. Yoga is a great training ground for learning how to relate to life's exigencies: it enables you to use maximally the learning possibilities that come to you.

As you do your yoga practices you will probably notice a gentle, natural progress in the direction of living in accordance with the yamas: non-injury, truthfulness, non-theft, spiritual conduct, non-greed. It is easier and more comfortable to do so. You might want to evaluate yourself occasionally as to the progress you are making. An easy way to do that is to consider each yama briefly and rate yourself on a scale from 1 to 10. It is also useful to record your score in your journal or other personal information file. Having done that, simply look at the score. Be gentle with yourself. It is important to be aware of your development, but still to let it take its own natural course.

Now let's look at the niyamas or observances.

4

Niyamas: Things to Do

Niyamas – five observances performed continually by all serious aspirants of Yoga. They are: physical and internal purity, contentment with one's material state, austerity, study of Yoga psychology and books of Self-knowledge, and Self-surrender to the divine object of meditation.

Rammurti S. Mishra, M.A., M.D.

Yoga has been and will be the main focus in my life. I try to make its principles the undercurrent of everything I do. In addition to developing physical equilibrium through asanas and meditation, I rely a great deal on the inspiration received from reading the divine wisdom books, such as the *Bhagavad Gita*, Patanjali's *Yoga Sutras*, etc. In addition, I reflect on the Buddha's teachings for an understanding of this scientific world we live in and Christ's teaching for fulfilling personal relationships in love.

Altogether, as the days go by I feel a greater and greater sense of *center*. Thanks to yoga I no longer fling myself helplessly from extreme to extreme. And in growing awareness and sensitivity, I find a growing freedom. To me, this is what life is mainly about!

Yoga student

The niyamas or observances are things to remember to do. They include: (a) cleanliness, (b) contentment, (c) austerity, (d) self-study, and (e) attentiveness to God or the All of existence. As we discuss them, we will discuss both the ethical and physiological aspects.

Cleanliness

Here the old expression, "cleanliness is next to Godliness," has new meaning. It must be viewed in context of how cleanliness contributes to one's peace of mind. Cleanliness soothes. It contributes to a relaxed physiology. When you live in a jumble of objects, you feel anxious, confused, unsettled. You feel out of touch with things when you need them.

We might look at the concept of entropy in the universe: disorder in the universe or the unavailable energy in a thermodynamic system. This concept derives from the laws of thermodynamics. Theoretically, the universe ends when there is maximum disorder. How this could be true is hard to imagine. All situations begin with order; all situations gradually degenerate. Life contributes negative entropy—order in the universe. On a more gross level, living in disorder contributes to disordered consciousness.

We live in the midst of environmental stimulation. If we are aware of stimulation, even minimally, then it stimulates our nervous systems. An increase in activity of bodily systems is caused by our response to this stimulation. Your mind, being highly responsive, repeatedly notices a disordered environment. In the stimulus array there is a lack of symmetry. Alert, you notice the changes in the pattern. Why? Repeatedly signaling you, the array of objects shows you that it is out of kilter. It demands to be taken care of.

There is also the factor of environmental stimulation. When you live in disorder, that is what is suggested to your nervous system: a disordered pattern. Your environment presents a pattern which you mirror with your consciousness. From increased order within yourself comes increased order in your environment, and vice versa.

One way to increase order within yourself is to meditate; there are others ways. The more you become internally focused and unified through your yoga practice, the more it becomes helpful to order your environment. Your environment will begin to mirror your inner calm. This internal-external feedback—your perceptions coloring your experiences—will enable you to move more and more in the direction of cleanliness.

Contentment

This niyama of contentment refers to acceptance of situations, to relating to situations without effort. Events are the results of past actions; past actions are the results of your prior perceptions. Therefore, accept and learn from these events.

Do you know people who live in discontent? They are not satisfied with anything; they spend long hours discussing how awful everything is. They begin with themselves. Then they extend to the community. Finally, they discuss the world. They sit there, unable to act. They cannot right the wrongs they perceive. As they talk, they generate physiological changes in their own bodies, and in the bodies of those who listen to them. They live and relive the unfortunate aspects of life. They create a physiological state with their attitudes. That state breeds more of the same perceptions.

There is much that needs to be changed in the world, I am not denying that. You must actively move to help change the human condition. Otherwise, you—constantly frustrated and agonizing—will stew in the juices of your discontent. This only makes it worse.

Through yoga practice, you will begin to change your physiological state. You will be more likely to dwell on that with which you are contented, to be motivated to help change what you are able to change, and to begin to change the subject every time you notice you've begun the broken record of discontent. You will shift over to a more parasympathetic nervous system balance, to relaxation. As you shift, you will notice that your moods are more pleasant.

Austerity

The term "austerity" reminds one of the hair shirts worn in the Middle Ages or of fakirs lying on beds of nails. In reality, austerity, or living in severe conditions, represents a simplified life and freedom from distractions. These distractions, which prevent you from achieving and maintaining higher states of consciousness, are another form of excess baggage. In ancient times, it was considered necessary to weaken the body's hold on the soul. It was thought that without the body to hold it back, the soul was free.

What is meant here, actually, is balanced bodily conditioning. When you live more simply and stringently, new internal experiences are possible. These new, internal experiences are not blocked by outside sensory input. The person who moves toward the austere life is not leaving a desired experience behind, but choosing a more desired experience. Such a path of austerity is beautiful for those who choose it. Turning down the thermostat in your house so that your own body heat will be intensified is one example. The experiencing of internal hallucinations or visions that come with prolonged sensory deprivation is another.

Self-Study

Self-study refers to the study of the larger Self. From this need comes the inclusion of daily study of sacred literature, from any tradition. Examples include the *Bhagavad-Gita*, the *Yoga Sutras*, the *Upanishads*, the *Bible*, Sufi literature, and so forth. Not only does self-study include reading the sacred literature, but also the study of one's deeper Self, one's own divine nature.

Reading from the sacred literature accomplishes several things, as well as reminding you of the larger reality. It helps you set the tone for the day; it helps you return to your more relaxed state.

Attentiveness to God

Let us expand our understanding of this niyama. The use of yoga to develop physical culture is one approach to yogic development; the use of yoga to develop spiritual culture, another. This niyama especially relates to the latter approach. We will expand the word God to include the Absolute, all that is, cosmic consciousness, the fabric of existence, or the ground of Being—whatever you use as a term for the larger reality. This niyama refers to maintaining, as much as possible, an awareness of the larger reality, and avoiding being caught in a limited view of one's self, one's situation, or one's life.

Finding God in everything you see and experience enables you to change the way you understand situations. You experience a changed understanding, an acceptance of situations, not necessarily a change in the situations themselves. This leads to an increase in a sense of union with existence.

As you do your yoga practice over time, you will notice changes in the direction of living more in accordance with the yamas and niyamas. You might also want to evaluate your progress toward the niyamas in the same way you evaluated the yamas. Consider each niyama briefly and rate yourself on a scale from 1 to 10 as to the degree to which you included that niyama in your daily schedule. Perhaps it would be simply a checklist which you would use daily or periodically. Now that we have looked at the yamas and niyamas as a behavioral context or lifestyle, let's begin our exploration of the somatic approach to the asanas or physical postures.

PART TWO

The Body in Somatic Yoga

5

Asanas: What to Do

Posture becomes firm and relaxed through control of the natural tendencies of the body, and through meditation on the infinite.

Patanjali

I've enjoyed practicing yoga because I'm constantly noticing changes and improvements in the way I feel. Mostly I enjoy hatha yoga and doing the meditations, although I am beginning to realize the importance of doing prana.

Yoga student

That there are so many yoga postures – 84,000 variations, plus or minus – is a tribute to human ingenuity. They are varied, but they lead to the same goal. If you are overwhelmed by the variety, you can begin with a basic set of postures. This basic set can provide you with a solid starting point for developing your own repertoire of yoga postures. The basic set includes these postures: corpse, legs up position, half shoulderstand, shoulderstand, fish, plough, cobra, locust, bow, spinal twist, yoga mudra, head-to-knee pose, stork, tree, and headstand.

Not only should you be concerned with doing the posture, but with *how* you are doing the posture. The next concern is what you are doing with your mind – the monkey of the mind. Your body may be stilled, but your attention, still moving. Getting your mind together with your body is a little like training a horse: it must be done in easy stages. From easy, repeated practice sessions comes a gradual moving together in time of your mental and physical activities. At first there are brief moments of integration or union, which lead to longer periods. Accomplished yogis are able to maintain that state permanently. But do not let that concern you now.

Counting and saying a mantra, visualizing the posture and attending to movements, doing the corpse and deep breathing afterwards are all ways of maximizing the effects of each posture. Counting enables you to hold your attention on the posture and measure the amount of time you maintain the posture and move it toward becoming a meditation posture. Counting—difficult at the beginning—becomes, with practice, as natural as breathing.

An exercise, a meditation practice, a relaxant—each posture has directions like a recipe (pinch of this, a dash of that; hold it this long, breathe this way, etc.). The recipe includes two directions: how to breathe and how long to hold the posture. If you hold the posture too long, if you do not breathe properly, if you do not attend to what you are doing, then you will have only some of the benefits of having done the posture. For each stage in your development there are benefits which will be present at that time, but not later. Who would want to miss them?

During all postures, it is helpful to do the yoga or Om-count. Om-1, Om-2, Om-3, and so forth, said sub-vocally, enables you to focus your attention on what you are doing. This is a unification experience. The Om-count facilitates your practice, insuring greater attention, measuring the amount of time in the posture, and moving you toward a more meditative experience. You can make progress in your yogic development, but only at the rate that is appropriate for you (your temperament, body type, lifestyle, destiny). Too much would throw you into a stress state; too little would leave you in a non-yogic state.

Somatic yoga uses the following principles to facilitate the learning and optimizing of the yogic experience: repetition, comfort and pleasure, self-sensing, moving out of gravity, learning slowly, awareness focussed on movement, internal visualization of movement, and unification of the first and third-person perspectives.

Repetition

Somatic yoga recognizes the value of the repetition of stimuli that is a part of yoga practice. This repetition enables you gradually to improve the movements by successive approximations of the completed posture. Yoga is an experience of getting past the boredom state to the stage of greater complexity of perception within the narrowed perceptual field. When you become restless and wish to move around, but don't, there is frequently a shift in your level of consciousness due to the inhibition of the tendency to deploy your attention elsewhere.

Comfort and Pleasure

Somatic yoga encourages the practitioner gradually to extend his practice as it becomes easier. One way you can do this is to wait until you spontaneously find yourself holding a posture longer before you set a different time frame. Somatic yoga emphasizes making your yoga practice as easy and effortless as possible. The purpose of this is to keep the general tone of the body within a parasympathetic nervous system dominance. Somatic yoga does not move to extremes, but tries to stay with what is easy and natural for the person. The purpose for this is again to avoid throwing the person into the orienting reflex and sympathetic nervous system response (the "fight or flight" response), with its biochemical changes.

Somatic yoga also emphasizes the pleasantness of the experience. Yoga, from time to time, speaks of bliss consciousness or *ananda*, that is, joy. One of the starting places for the experience of joy is in the body's experience of pleasure in the stretching and relaxation of various parts. As the individual does his practice, he is encouraged to experience and enhance the pleasurable sensations of self-sensing during and after yoga practice. He learns to appreciate the experience of the sensory feedback, and perhaps also the production of endorphins and other biochemical products that accompany pleasure.

Self-Sensing: The Motor-Sensory Loop

In somatic yoga, there is an emphasis on both sides of the sensorimotor loop. As the person does the posture, both while moving into the posture and afterwards, he is sensing the effects, the physiological feedback cues of movement. This is picked up by sensing the changes in the bodily area, subtle vibrations, feelings of greater awareness or aliveness in the area.

Differatiation – Integration = Organization

In somatic yoga there is an emphasis on differentiating between certain movements and positions, focusing on them, being aware of them, and holding the position for an extended period of time. These movements and postures are removed from the ordinary flow of movements and deliberately performed. Then, when you go about your business during the day, you will be more ready to use your body flexibly and fully for the exercises and movements that are necessary. You also will have less restriction of movement, because your body has already enlivened the neural circuits and pathways leading to the muscles involved. In that way, you first differentiate the movement from others, and then, as you go about your everyday business, you integrate the isolated practice into the total organization of your movements.

Speaking of organization, somatic yoga emphasizes being fully aware of one's unified body/mind during all activities of the day. Since the body will be organizing itself more efficiently for the actions that it takes, you are also encouraged to be more aware of the integrated action at the same time. This awareness is very difficult to maintain, but it can become increasingly habitual for you as you practice it.

Moving Out of Gravity

There are several ways in which somatic yoga uses a change in your relationship to gravity. One of the ways is that many of the movements and postures are done while lying on the floor or close to the floor. Also, many of the postures reverse the body's position in the earth's gravitational field. When you are lying down, without the strain and activating aspects of being upright in gravity, it is possible to be more relaxed and to have your mind free for reflection and the absorption of directions, information, and insights that well up from within your mind.

Learn Slowly/Move Slowly

In somatic yoga it is considered important to move very slowly with as much awareness as possible. It is important to learn the postures and other practices very slowly, proceeding at your own rate. Make sure that you always feel comfortable with where you are in your development. Move very slowly into each posture or practice.

Awareness While Moving

As demonstrated by Moshe Feldenkrais (1972) and others, it is extremely important in somatic yoga or any other activity to be as sharply aware as possible of each movement of the body during the posture or practice. This is of cardinal importance. You must move slowly enough to be able to remain aware, mindful, throughout the movement. If the teacher or a taped instruction gives the directions, the guide can be used to help you remember to keep your attention on each aspect of the movement and the body's organization of itself as it carries out the movement. When you are doing your yoga practice alone, you will have to remember constantly to return your attention to your practice. If a teacher is guiding you, you can become more relaxed because you are not in executive control, making the decisions about where you should place your attention next, and so forth. This allows your mind to be freer and to have more of the areas of the brain that are particularly important unimpeded by activation of other brain areas.

Internal Visualization

Somatic yoga uses internal visualization to facilitate each posture. Internal visualization of the posture makes it easier to learn at the beginning. It enables your central nervous system to get a complete picture of where it is going. Do not launch abruptly into the posture, but fully prepare yourself in advance. Later, after you have learned the posture, continue to visualize it before doing it in order to facilitate the assumption and maintenance of the posture.

Therefore, each time we do a posture in somatic yoga, we first visualize ourselves doing the posture. When we move slowly into the posture, remaining mindful of each of the movements as the body organizes itself to accomplish the posture. We hold the posture for the recommended length of time and the length of time which suits our present level of development. We do the yoga count while maintaining the posture so that we can stay attentive, make it a meditative experience, and measure the amount of time that we maintain the posture. Then we come slowly out of the posture, again trying to stay as mindful of each movement as possible.

After the posture we take the corpse position for a minute of deep breathing. While lying there, we are aware of the sensory sensations that are present throughout our bodies. While doing the posture, there is activity of the motor cortex; while doing the corpse, we pay attention to the after-effect of the motor activity, which is signaled by activity of the sensory cortex. This enables us to get full benefit from the posture, rather than moving quickly toward the the next posture, which competes with the sensory cortex for neural activation.

The Samyama of Asanas

Samyama is a high state of concentration which combines the three practices—concentration, meditation, and unification or absorption into the object of attention—into a single practice. In somatic yoga, the asanas are done in the samyama fashion. The first stage includes focusing your attention (concentration) while achieving the posture. The second stage includes the repeated neuromuscular impulses needed to maintain the posture—the meditative experience. The third stage includes the awareness of the sensations generated before, during, and after the posture.

An important practice in yoga is to move toward identification with supreme consciousness or the ultimate. This will enable you to realize that you are more than the limitations of your body and your personality. The release from the heaviness of one's individual life is very helpful in gaining some peace. It is very valuable to have the flexibility to focus on one's individual life, and also to be able to disconnect and feel more detached. The more you practice this wider identification, the easier it gets. How can you achieve it? A recipe for practicing this wider identification is the following: place your attention on supreme consciousness; suggest that you are identified with it, then feel that you have lost the awareness of your body. Finally, feel that you have identified with supreme consciousness. If your mind wanders, bring it back to focus on supreme consciousness.

Asana As Meditation

An asana is a bodily aid to concentration. Postures should accomplish the following things (Mishra, 1959, p. 158):

1. "A posture should relax the body and the mind." Here we have a necessity to relax the body from its muscular and biochemical tensions. We must also deliberately free the mind from its preoccupations with the body. Doing the physical posture will help with clearing the mind.

2. "It should give strength to the body and the mind." This refers to strengthening the muscles and the neural circuits that enable both to function effectively.

3. "It should remove all mental and physical burdens, anxieties, and diseases." As we let go of the physical and mental constrictions, we cease to perpetuate the biochemical states and imbalances that support anxieties and provide a fertile field for disease.

4. "A posture should help [us] to forget the feeling of the body

so that consciousness may identify itself with supreme consciousness." If a posture is balanced and comfortable enough, it will free the consciousness to remember its relationship with supreme consciousness.

5. "A posture should give cultural and therapeutic advantages." This refers to the physical culture and health benefits of doing yoga postures.

6. "A posture should be uninterrupted, firm, and easy." This means that extreme postures should not be used for concentration. The goal of raja yoga is to facilitate concentration by facilitating the state of consciousness conducive to concentration.

Mishra (1959) reminds us that the later stages of yoga are physically quite demanding. There is a great need at that time for physical strength and endurance. If the body is not fully trained and prepared, samadhi will not be possible. The mind can move toward the higher stages, but not achieve them. A strenuous spiritual life — an ecstatic state — is very hard on the body. The body must achieve the most perfect development and control possible. This is aided by the use of the postures.

Mishra says that "perfection of the body consists of beauty, grace, strength, and adamantine hardness" (1959, p. 159). Adamantine is a very hard stone. If you consistently practice yoga, then the soma (living body) becomes its uniquely beautiful self. It is marvelous to observe the process of the individual developing his or her unique beauty: the body and movements become more graceful, smooth, and intelligent. A quiet strength develops. There is a sturdiness that is the preparation for the rigors of spiritual life.

The postures are a preparation for yoga or union, not ends in themselves. The mind and body are trained by the asanas toward spiritual development. The postures should give you a spiritual boost; you should feel a greater liveliness in your body.

Yoga sees the body and mind as interrelated. Neither can function effectively if the other is not functioning well. Yoga provides exercises for both, with the goal of achieving psychophysiological equilibrium. It is felt that consciousness is developed through perfection of the body and mind. How does this happen? Mishra (1959) says that due to our many incarnations we have forgotten our true nature, and that we feel our Self and consciousness to be limited by our bodies. Through the practice of yoga we begin to remember. We lose the sense of finiteness because the Self is infinite. Yoga is a process of de-hypnotism, and through concentration, meditation, and unification we can come to realize our true nature. Omnipresence, omnipotence, and omniscience—all are qualities of the Self.

Reminders

From our increasing ability to relax comes an increase in many of the benefits of yoga. So simple! The state of relaxation, you will find, enables you to keep your mind on what you're doing. As you are able to keep your mind on what you are doing, you will be able to integrate your movement fully with your awareness. Yoga training is an evolving process; it entails successive approximations of the postures until you are able to perfect them. The trick is to go as far with the posture as you can without strain; go as far as you can, with patience. Experiencing, perceiving, and learning, you will have a before-and-after picture of your yogic development. Each stage in your development is important in its own right.

How do we begin? I usually introduce each posture with a demonstration of the posture. The posture is held for about 10 seconds so that a visual image may be formed by the observer. Each observer closes his eyes and revisualizes the posture for about 10 seconds. The visualization being completed, he then attempts the posture. In future classes he will repeat this process of visualizing the posture for about 10 seconds before doing it. The visualization process—focusing and relaxing—greatly facilitates yogic practice and development.

Not only do we visualize each posture before we do it, but we also pause after each posture to do the corpse pose. The corpse pose is the simplest. When we move too quickly from one activity to another, when we do not pause to recover from the previous activity, when we do not collect our thoughts in between, we do not make maximum use of the original activity. The corpse pose in this case has two benefits: it allows a minute for relaxation and allows us to sense the effects of the previous posture. To do the posture and miss the after-effects is to miss many of the benefits of the posture. Relaxing and sensing are both parts of the stage that follows each posture.

As we do the corpse, we do a minute of deep breathing. For every four seconds we have inhaled, we exhale for an equal amount of time. With this diaphragmatic breathing, I usually count to 64 using the Om count. This is a little more than one minute in duration.

You will develop in yoga what you intend to develop. The ancient, simple, transcendent effects are not just for the talented few. All who practice, depending on the quality and quantity of the practice, will have results. Knowing yoga well, you will find yourself using it consciously and unconsciously in your everyday life. One way to make full use of your yoga practice is to write about it: write down the insights that come to you during or after yoga practice. From writing in your yoga journal comes awareness you may not even know you have until you begin to write.

General Steps for Somatic Yoga Postures

1. Visualize the posture for 10 Oms.

2. Move slowly into the posture. Take about 10 Oms to get into it.

3. Do the Om-count while holding the posture; keep your attention on the posture.

4. Follow the appropriate breath pattern for that posture.

5. Come slowly out of the posture. Take about 10 Oms.

6. Take the corpse position. Do deep breathing for about one minute or 60 Oms.

7. During that time, be aware. Practice self-sensing. Scan your

body for the after-effects of having done the posture: proprioceptive sensations, heat changes, differences in body position, feelings of relaxation.

    8. Visualize the next posture.

The following postures are presented as a basic set which is
the core of somatic yoga: corpse, legs up position, half shoulderstand, shoulderstand, fish, plough, cobra, locust, bow, spinal
twist, yoga mudra, head-to-knee pose, stork, tree, and headstand. Others may be added for variety and special purposes. A
possible organization for your yoga session is presented at the end
of the chapter.

The Corpse (Figure 5.1)

The corpse is the easist of the yoga postures. Lie on the floor with
your legs outstretched, feet about 20 inches apart, hands about 10
inches from your sides, palms up. Find a comfortable position
with your body as symmetrical as possible. Make sure your back
is as relaxed as possible. Be careful that it is not unconsciously
arched. Wiggle your feet and hands and roll your head slightly to
make sure that you are relaxed.

    Do a minute of deep breathing when doing the corpse position
between postures. This supplies the body with plenty of oxygen,
encourages relaxation, and enables you to practice self-sensing. A
subtle ability, self-sensing enables you to be aware of the effects of
the postures so that you can get maxium benefit from them. I have
used the analogy that doing the posture is like peddling a 10-
speed bicycle: you coast on the momentum while doing the
corpse. Another analogy that has been helpful is to consider your
physiological state as being like a lake into which a pebble has
been dropped. It is valuable to wait after each posture to allow the
ripples to complete their expansion outward before dropping
another pebble.

    The minute of deep breathing has abdominal breathing as its
goal. With four Oms inhaling and four Oms exhaling, count to 64.

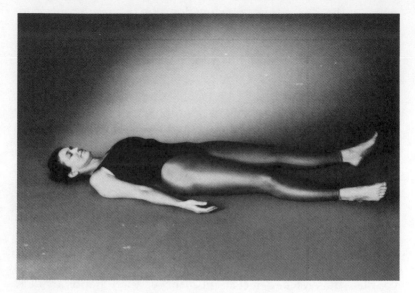

FIGURE 5.1 The Corpse

Each count should be about one second. It is helpful to time your-self at some point to see what the frequency of one Om per second feels like. Breathe in and out quietly and easily. It should not be forced.

The corpse posture is said to relax the mind and body. The nerves and muscles are soothed, rested, restored. Ordinarily when we sleep, we do not remain relaxed but go through various neuromuscular experiences. With the corpse position you delib-erately, consciously remain relaxed for a given period of time. It is said that venous blood returns more easily to the heart, and that the biochemical effects of fatigue are removed through this pos-ture. It has been shown to reduce high blood pressure (Patel, 1975; Patel, 1973; Patel & North, 1975). It helps reduce anxiety and ner-vousness. This state, a reduction in muscle tone and a shift toward the parasympathetic nervous system, includes biochemistry that is less contributory to the anxiety response.

Legs Up Position (Figure 5.2)

Lie on the floor in the corpse position. Bend your knees and slowly raise your feet toward the ceiling. Straighten your legs so that they are perpendicular to the floor. Your arms rest on the floor beside your body; hands palms down. Take about 10 seconds to assume the position. Breathe as regularly as possible while in the position. In the beginning, hold the position for about 20 seconds. Later you will extend the time that you hold the position until you are able to maintain it comfortably for about one minute. When you are ready to come out of the position, bend your knees. Bring your feet slowly down to the floor. Then slide your feet away from you along the floor. Finally, your legs rest gently on the floor. You are again in the corpse position.

Shoulderstand (Figure 5.3)

Stately and poised, the shoulderstand is also referred to as the candle. It is said to facilitate metabolism through stimulation of the thyroid. It is basically a simple pose, but must be moved into gradually. Reversing the flow of gravity through the body, sending increased nutrition to the face and brain, helping with varicose veins, chest development and strengthening shoulders — these are many of the reasons why it is such a valued pose.

Beginning a new posture is essentially a sympathetic nervous system activity. At this point you will not want to hold the position too long — too long would produce strain. Gradually, you will be able to extend the amount of time from the initial 20 seconds (or 20 Oms) to a minute or several minutes. When we first learn a behavior there is total brain activation; later, less brain activity is present; still later, only the area of the brain required for the activity shows any activation.

The shoulderstand is a very complete posture. Valued next to the headstand, it is similar in terms of its overall benefits. Begin by looking at the picture of the shoulderstand for ten Oms. Close your eyes and see the posture in your mind's eye for 10 Oms.

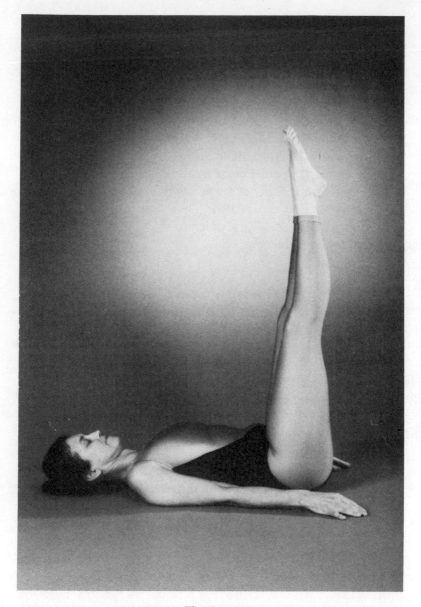

FIGURE 5.2 The Legs Up Position

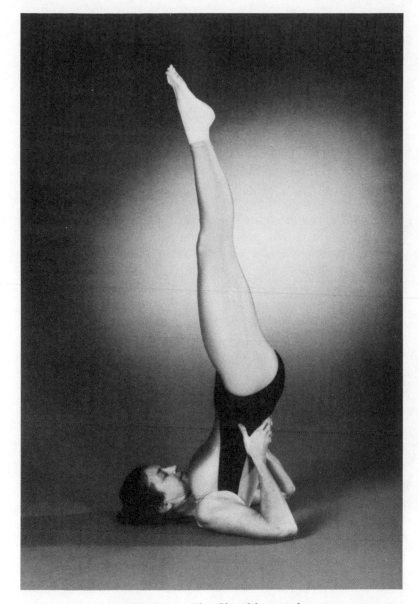

FIGURE 5.3 The Shoulderstand

When you have finished, take the corpse position and relax for a moment. With your arms remaining on the floor, slowly bend your knees. Move them toward your chest. Lift your knees higher, round your back, and lift your bottom off the ground. Extend your legs slowly toward the ceiling. Bend your elbows and support your back with your hands. Move your torso as far forward as possible. It should be perpendicular to the floor. Your chin should rest on your chest. Keep your eyes open. Focus them on the center of your torso. Breathe as regularly as possible. Remain in the posture for 20 Oms. In subsequent yoga sessions, add 30 Oms per week until you can maintain the posture comfortably for three minutes. When you are ready to come out of the posture, bend your knees and round your back. As your feet reach the floor, slide them slowly out until you are again in the corpse position. Remain there for one minute, breathing deeply and sensing after-effects of the posture.

The after-effects may be tingling sensations, temperature changes, a feeling of having stretched a muscle group, or a greater awareness of the area.

The shoulderstand, due to its focus of pressure and attention on the throat region, is said to stimulate the thyroid. When the thyroid is functioning effectively, the entire body is in a healthier state. The shoulderstand is said to aid in keeping the sexual systems of both sexes in good condition. This is particularly true with such conditions as displaced uterus. The shoulderstand helps with dyspepsia, which is the result of impaired digestive processes. This posture helps relieve constipation also. Hernias can sometimes be relieved. Visceroptosis is a condition marked by a dropping of the viscera or internal organs. Many people, as they get older, have postural difficulties which leave their internal organs with insufficient skeletal-muscular support. The shoulderstand does two things to help this condition: it benefits abdominal muscles and the function of internal organs in that region.

One version of the advanced shoulderstand is done with the arms flat on the floor; a more advanced version is done with arms remaining at the sides. As you do these you will discover an amazing fact: you are holding the posture by balance alone. Poised, your head and shoulders make a tripod.

As always, assume the corpse position after each posture. Allow the somatic sensations to flow; remain relaxed and aware. Do the four count deep breathing (four Oms inhale; four Oms exhale) for about one minute.

Half Shoulderstand (Figure 5.4)

The half shoulderstand is a modification of the shoulderstand and is somewhat more difficult to execute for the beginner. Bottom and hands, neck and chin, breath and sight facilitate the flow of stimulation to areas of the brain involved with extrasensory perception (it is said). The effect of the position is to send impulses from the vestibular system to the cerebellum and reticular activating system. Proprioceptors also signal the position of the body in space.

The Fish (Figure 5.5)

It is good to follow the shoulderstand with the fish pose. From observing the illustration, you can see that in the fish pose the neck is bent in the opposite direction from the way it is bent in the shoulderstand. If you do the shoulderstand effectively, if you remain aware, if you have savored the experience, then the fish will bring fresh input to your nervous system. This helps to facilitate the effect of the previous posture.

The beginning fish is achieved with your legs stretched out in front of you. Relaxed and attentive, place your elbow on the ground behind you. Gently lean down on the other elbow and ease your head down to the floor behind you. From that position, slowly look toward the floor behind you. Relax. Hold that pose for 20 Oms. In each successive yoga session, extend the time by abut 30 Oms—three minutes is the recommended maximum extension of the pose. As soon as you have assumed the posture, remember to relax your entire body and breathe regularly. Be aware of the sensations of that posture.

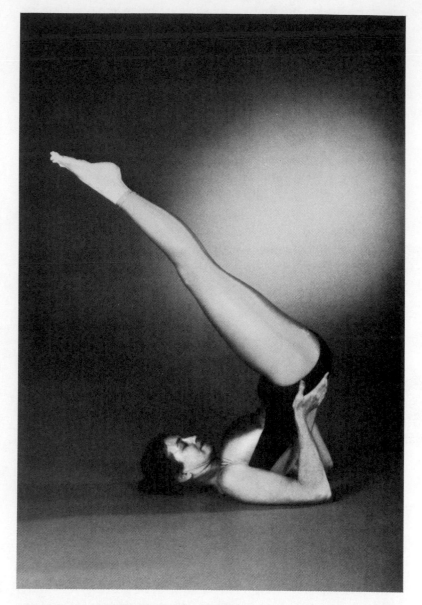

FIGURE 5.4 The Half Shoulderstand

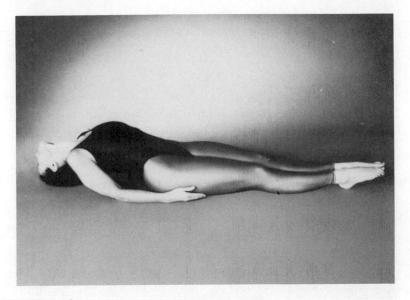

FIGURE 5.5 The Fish

When I first began to do the fish, it was my least favorite posture. Not only did I not enjoy it, I did not appreciate its benefits. Then one day, about six months later, I noticed that I felt like I was relaxing and floating. It was delicious.

The advanced fish is done from the lotus position. How this is done may seem mysterious to you at first. As you go into the posture, be sure you support yourself on one elbow so that your back will not be strained by the unsupported arch. If you are not careful, you will accentuate the hyperextension of your back. Position your head on the floor as in the beginning fish; hook your fingers around your big toes.

The fish pose is said to help the back, chest, and neck. The muscles of the trapezius are contracted, while the flexors of the chest are relaxed. This is a valuable alteration of the usual condition and helps release them for greater comfort. It slows down abdominal and sexual system degeneration.

It has been said that the fish will enable you to survive in the water for a long time. I have tried it in the water; I sink. Of course,

I cannot float under any circumstances. I swim like a fish, but I float like a sinker. I have no doubt that others have achieved it. Try it in shallow water first.

The Plough (Figure 5.6)

The plough position begins from the supine position. Slowly bend your knees. Bring them up toward your chest. Your arms— supporters—remain on the floor to assist in moving your legs slowly over your head. (The plough can be done with your arms extended toward your feet or in the opposite direction.) Move slowly. Your flexibility permitting, make the entire movement slow and deliberate. Extend your legs behind you until your toes touch the floor behind your head. Then straighten your knees. Gradually relax in the posture. Keep your eyes open. How long should you hold it? In the beginning, remain in the posture for 20 Oms. In later sessions, extend the time you hold the posture until you can remain in it for four minutes without strain. Your chin should eventually rest on your chest.

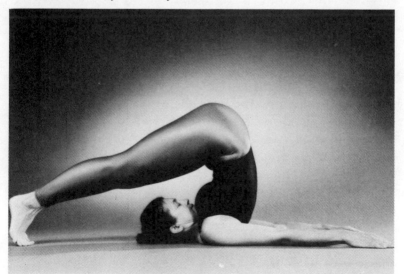

FIGURE 5.6 The Plough

When you first attempt the plough, you will probably find yourself stiffer than you would like to be. Achieving it will seem impossible. If you cannot touch the floor, bring your feet as close to the floor as you can comfortably. Hold them there for 20 Oms; at a later date you will find yourself more able to complete the posture as pictured. Be gentle with yourself, be content with each stage of your development.

Breathe as gently and regularly as you can. Cramped by the extreme bend in your neck, this will not be easy. It is also more difficult to do the plough in the morning than in the evening. This is one of the examples of the benefits of the warm-up movements: the plough will come more easily after warm-ups.

The plough pose is said to relieve joint diseases. This could be the effect of reducing the tension on arthritic pained joints. The plough also helps to tone up the abdominal and chest muscles and enables the spine to be more elastic. Because of the increased muscle tone, the standing posture of the person who practices the plough will be improved. Also, it is thought that the plough stimulates the thyroid. When the thyroid functions better, the whole body is healthier.

The Cobra (Figure 5.7)

The cobra follows the plough because it involves an opposing movement of the spine. You begin the posture from the prone position (belly down) with your legs extended and feet together. Place your palms down, beside your shoulders. Inhale and gradually lift your chest from the ground. Feel as though your spine is lifting segment by segment. Feel as though your inhaling is what lifts you from the ground. Look toward the ceiling with your eyes open.

Hold your breath in the position for about 10 Oms. Relax. Exhale, slowly, as you come out of the position. Inhale again as you resume the position—the hooded cobra. This kind of mindfulness will help you get the most from the posture. Take about

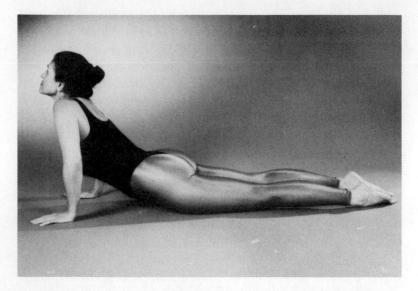

FIGURE 5.7 The Cobra

10 Oms to get into the position and 10 Oms to get out of it. Repeat the posture about three times.

The cobra pose strengthens the back by giving the muscles of the back an opportunity to contract. This is particularly true of the muscles of the lower back—the extensor muscles. At the same time, the abdominal muscles are relaxed. You do not want to end with the cobra pose without some posture or movement that contracts the abdominal muscles and relaxes the lower back. If you did, it would leave you with a hyperextended back and lead to further tightness in your lower back.

The cobra pose can help reposition spinal column displacements in certain conditions. The sympathetic and parasympathetic nervous systems are said to be stimulated by the cobra. The sympathetic nervous system has its pathway along the spinal column; the parasympathetic nervous system, from the cervical and caudal ends of the spinal column. It is said that indigestion and flatulence are relieved through this pose. The greater the shift to the parasympathetic nervous system, the more digestion will be aided.

The Half Locust (Figure 5.8)

The half locust is one of the postures done from the prone position. Your head rests on your chin, arms by your sides, palms on the floor. Extend one leg in the air as far as possible behind you. Inhale while going into the position, exhale as you come out. Hold the position for about 10 Oms. Extend the legs one at a time from side to side 3 to 7 times.

As you hold postures for extended time periods, there are new effects. Relaxation, calmness, ease—all these are experienced as the effort of achieving the position is surmounted.

The locust pose is said to benefit the pelvic region. The locust pose also tones up abdominal muscles and helps improve circulation to the legs.

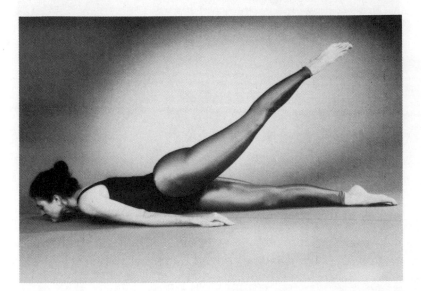

FIGURE 5.8 The Half Locust

The Bow (Figure 5.9)

The bow begins from the prone position. Bend your knees so that your lower legs are at right angles to your torso. Reach one arm behind you and grasp your ankle. Now reach the other arm around to grasp the other ankle. You are now a relaxed bow, as in an archer's bow. Pull the bow, your body, taut by pulling against yourself. Exhale as you go into the complete position. Arch. Hold your breath out for about 10 Oms. From this position, look toward the ceiling. Inhale as you relax coming out of the position; exhale as you tighten the bow again. Repeat the alternating tension and relaxation 3 to 7 times.

The bow pose stretches the stomach muscles and the muscles in the hips. It will help to lessen curvature of the spine, if it is appropriate to the kind of curvature present; it will help eliminate gas. It also helps reduce stomach fat.

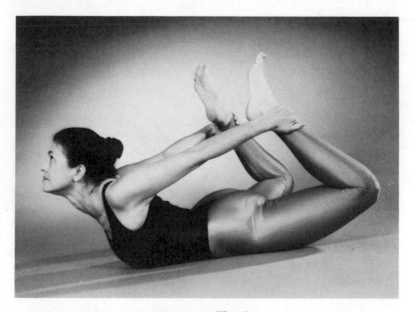

FIGURE 5.9 The Bow

The Spinal Twist (Figure 5.10)

The spinal twist is one of the more complex poses. Not only is it a stately pose, it offers delightful rewards once it is accomplished. It is beautiful to see an entire class doing it. How is it done? There are several variations of the spinal twist. Here is one of them.

Sit on the ground with both feet in front of you. Bend your knees slightly. Bring the heel of one foot under your bent knee to rest beside your bottom on the opposite side. Next bring the remaining heel to rest just to the other side of the knee in front of you. Twist your body around so that the opposite arm is draped over the up-turned knee. Curl it around to touch the opposite side of that instep. Then bring the other arm around your waist. Turn your head and eyes as far around as possible. Focus your eyes on a spot on the wall. Breathe as regularly as possible. Hold the position for about 20 Oms when you begin. Eventually you may want to hold it for 60 Oms—approximately a minute. Now slowly unwind. Return to your starting position. Repeat the posture on the opposite side.

The spinal twist is a posture that twists the spine in two directions. Because of that the spinal column is benefited, the sympathetic nervous system is also benefited. The muscles of the shoulders are massaged internally as are the muscles of the abdomen. Constipation is said to be relieved through practice of this posture, and indigestion is lessened. The liver, spleen, and kidneys are also said to be benefited.

Yoga Mudra (Figure 5.11)

The yoga mudra can be done from a cross-legged position or from the lotus position. In the lotus position you place the right foot on your left thigh near the torso. Then you bring your left foot up over your right knee until it rests on your right thigh near the torso. People vary as to how easy it is for them to do the lotus; some people do it quite easily, others have a great deal of difficulty with it.

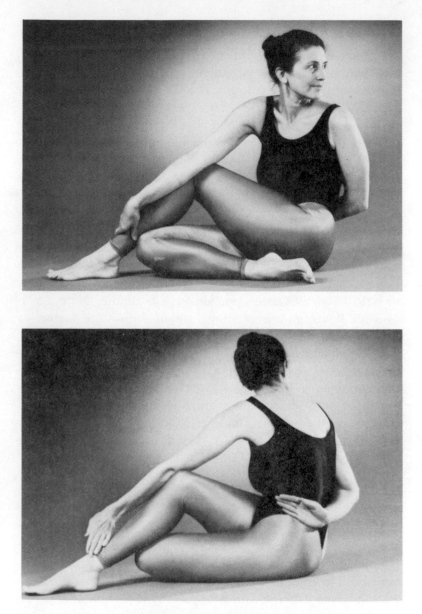

FIGURE 5.10 The Spinal Twist

Having assumed the lotus position or cross-legged position, bring your arms behind your back. Lace your fingers together. Straighten your arms behind you and raise them as high as you can. Exhale as you bend toward the floor in front of you. When

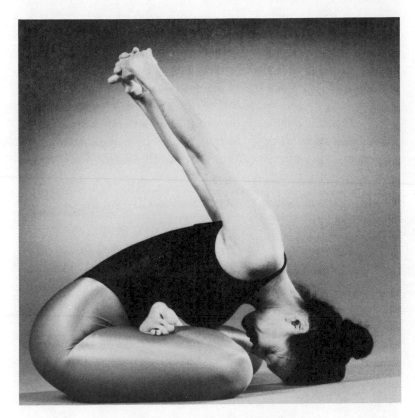

FIGURE 5.11 The Yoga Mudra

you reach the maximum forward bend (your forehead may be touching the floor), hold the position for about 20 seconds. Breathe as regularly as you can. At the end of that time sit up slowly. Take the corpse position for a minute of deep breathing.

The Head-to-knee Pose (Figure 5.12)

The head-to-knee pose was once considered a secret pose. It was never to be demonstrated in public, only in private. It was guarded not only because of its stimulation to the spinal cord, but because of its powerful effect on the kundalini. The kundalini pathway was said to parallel the spinal column.

The head-to-knee pose can be done sitting or standing. When done in a sitting position, you extend your legs out in front of you. Gracefully, lift your arms above your head. Exhale as you bring your arms down slowly, carefully, mindfully. Reach out with both

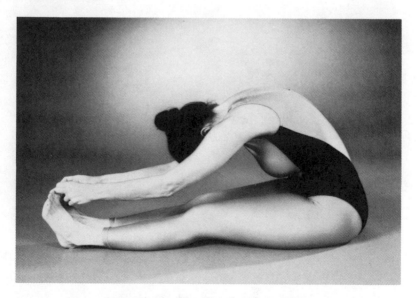

FIGURE 5.12 The Head-to-knee Pose

hand to grasp your big toes, but don't worry if you cannot touch them. If you cannot reach your toes or instep, simply grasp your ankles or calves. Gradually, bring your head down toward your knees. Keep your eyes open. Breathe as regularly as you can once you have achieved the position. Remember to notice where you may have become tense in achieving the position. Relax those areas. Go as far down as you can comfortably and hold it there. If you practice, if you relax, then as time goes on you will gradually become more flexible. At first, hold the pose for 20 Oms; gradually, with each practice session, extend the duration of the pose to about three minutes. Then relax back into the corpse position for one minute of deep breathing.

The head-to-knee standing pose starts from a standing position. Exhale as you bend over to grasp your knees from behind; your knees can be bent slightly. Blood pressure changes make it important not to hold the position too long. After 10 to 20 Oms at the most, resume the corpse position for relaxation, one minute of deep breathing and proprioceptive awareness.

The Stork (Figure 5.13)

The stork is the simplest of the standing poses. You begin by lifting one foot and resting it against your leg and continuing to hold your ankle. How to maintain your balance is a challenge. Fix your eyes on a spot on the floor. This will help you maintain your balance—loss of balance is signaled by the vestibular system. Your eyes are a valuable information feedback source for balancing.

This practice stimulates the vestibular system. The vestibular system—a complex associative system—plays an essential part in maintaining your balance. The vestibular system has connections with many areas of the brain. As you do this posture you will notice many movements of your body; these are designed to help you regain your balance. As you become more adept at this pose you will be steadier. Enjoy your initial wobbles. The posture can be used as a subtle way to wake yourself up; the nervous system's integrated involvement in balancing is quite alerting.

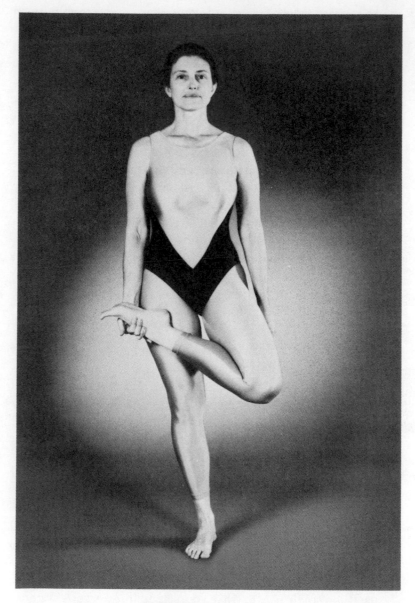

FIGURE 5.13 The Stork

The stork—stately, balanced on one leg—is one of the simplest standing poses. Feel like a stork. Gently pick up one foot, and gently hold it in front of the leg above the knee. Hold the bent leg by the ankle. After about 20 Oms, change sides. Remember to reverse sides on all bilateral postures.

The Tree (Figure 5.14)

I have become quite fond of the tree pose. I especially appreciate its capacity to make you feel "centered" and calm. Beginning with standing on both feet, slowly pick up one foot. With your other hand place your foot against your thigh. Now bring your hands over your head to rest palms together. With your eyes held steadily focused on a visual target, remain in that position for 20 Oms. Slowly lower your foot and hands. Now lift the other foot and repeat the posture.

The Headstand (Figure 5.15)

The headstand is the king of yoga postures. Depending upon the competency of the person doing the posture, it has a number of attributes claimed by numerous yogis: increased intelligence, prevention of greying and loss of hair through through increased circulation to the scalp, and reversal of the flow of gravity through the body. The headstand, the master posture, is very stimulating. By reversing the flow of gravity, it helps tone up all the systems. It has two effects on the consciousness—it will help you wake up in the morning and it will also help you go to sleep. Once when I was living alone, I had a great deal of trouble sleeping. I was under a lot of stress; I was in the process of finishing my doctorate. Each night I followed the same pattern: I would awaken every two hours all night long. I was unable to go back to sleep. So I began to do the headstand for a few seconds every time I woke up. It certainly saved my nights and subsequent days.

If you have any medical concerns, please consult your physician before attempting the headstand.

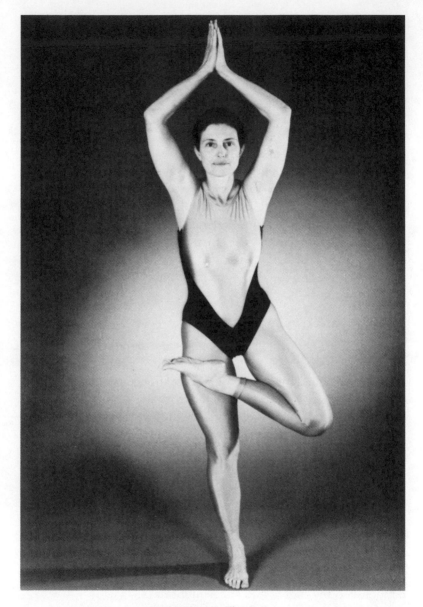

FIGURE 5.14 The Tree

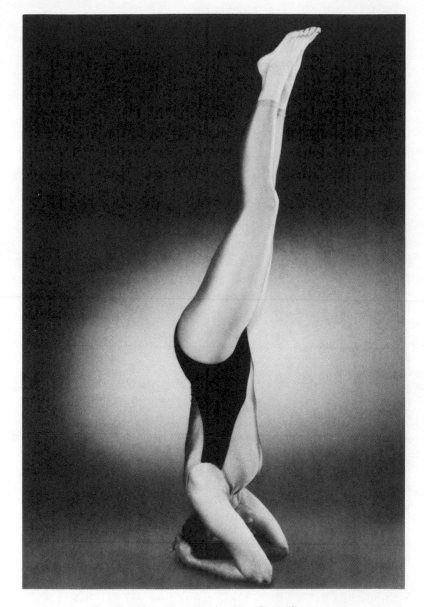

FIGURE 5.15 The Headstand

To learn the headstand, do not try to use a wall as some people do: it will only get in the way of discovering your own balance.

I remember how I felt when I first tried the headstand — scared. The headstand is said to increase your self-confidence and courage. Once you have conquered the headstand you will feel a new sense of self-confidence and courage.

Find a good spot to do the headstand. In fact, always do your yoga in a place where you have plenty of room. Use a blanket folded four times for padding. Lace your fingers together to form a cup. Place your hands palms up on the floor. Your elbows should be spread only the width of your head. It is a common mistake to let the elbows slide too far apart. You need to form a tripod with your head and arms. If the angle is too wide, there is less support for your body. For an example of this, try standing with your toes pointed out at 180° from each other (the second position in ballet). Therefore, it is best to begin with your elbows fairly close together. Some people can do the headstand with elbows apart using muscle strength. It is far better to hold the position through balance so that it is less of a strain.

The top of your head should be more or less on the floor. Firmly establish in your mind that, if you wish to come out of the position for any reason, you will come down in the same direction in which you went up. Erase from your mind the possibility that you can somersault backwards if you fail. Not only are you likely to hurt yourself if you allow that, but you also may cause yourself to panic. Simply maintain your balance and return to the floor when you feel ready.

Now walk toward your head with your knees bent. Stop when your back feels perpendicular to the floor. Tip your pelvis a bit more. Catch your balance with your legs bent. (You may wish to stop here for several sessions until your arms become strong enough to hold you. It is also helpful to have a friend spot for you until you easily know your way into the posture and out.) Ease your feet up toward the ceiling one at a time. Try to think of your legs being suspended from the ceiling by a string. Feel the easy flow of gravity. Keep your eyes open and fixed on a visual target.

Remember to relax when you have achieved the posture. Breathe easily. Do your Om count. Hold the pose for 20 Oms initially. You may wish to extend the time in later yoga sessions.

When it is time to come down from the headstand, simply bring one leg back down to the ground. Follow it gracefully with your other leg. Sit for seconds or minutes while your circulation reestablishes itself. You might even massage your face to increase facial circulation.

The headstand is said to increase the circulation of the blood to the brain. This change is not as great as it might seem. The cerebral blood supply is very well balanced against sudden large changes. The headstand is also said to stimulate the pineal body. The pineal body is a gland located just above the midbrain. Far-reaching in its effects, the headstand also stimulates the pituitary. The pituitary is located beneath the hypothalamus and is the master gland of the body. The headstand stimulates the cardiovascular system by changing the effect of the flow of gravity on the body. The digestive system seems to be stimulated, as does the entire nervous system. This is true because of the numerous efforts that the body needs to make in order to achieve the pose. It can help to remove some kinds of headaches. Dizziness, under certain circumstances, can be removed. It is said to help artereosclerosis by making the vessels more elastic. It helps improve memory. How? This is perhaps due to increased alertness. A certain level of alertness is necessary to be able to put information into memory storage, to retrieve memories. Intelligence – an elusive capacity – also seems to improve. This would be possible through increased nutrition and oxygen to the brain. Perhaps it has to do with the effects of stimulation on brain function, and results from the original experiences being dealt with more effectively. It is said to aid the function of the liver, spleen, and sexual system. Hernias can be relieved; viscerotopsis or displaced viscera, counteracted. So it is claimed. The headstand has been known to relieve some asthmatic discomforts.

In conclusion, the asanas are postures or a series of body positions designed to be held for periods of time. To derive maximum benefit from each is the goal. In raja yoga, the postures are used as meditative postures. A basic set of postures has been presented here, which includes the headstand, legs up position, half shoulderstand, corpse, plough, spinal twist, fish, bow, cobra, locust, yoga mudra, shoulderstand, head-to-knee pose, stork, and tree.

It is helpful to use the Om count to measure the time in each posture. Because this has a centering effect, it also helps make it a meditative experience. The asanas help prepare you for meditation, and for everyday life.

It would be valuable to remember to be aware of the benefits of these postures in a general way. Keeping in mind the beneficial aspects of the postures as you do them contributes to the overall effect of the practice.

Now that we have presented the basic set of postures, let's look at a possible organization for your yoga session. I would suggest that when you begin your yoga training, you do the first three postures for 20 Oms each. Then each week add the next posture. As you add each posture, begin with a 20 Om duration. For the postures that recommend extending the time progressively, add about 30 Oms each week until you reach the maximum time recommended for that posture or the maximum time that seems appropriate for you. This may also depend on how much time you have to devote to your yoga practice. A minimum of 30 Oms per posture is recommended if you are short of time. The longer you hold the posture comfortably, the greater will be the benefits. Remember, however, to observe the recommended time limits.

After you have gradually added postures, the structure of your yoga session might include the following:

Warm-up movements (3 minutes)

Asanas
    Legs up (1 minute)
    Half shoulderstand (40 seconds)
    Shoulderstand (3 minutes)
    Fish (3 minutes)
    Plough (3 minutes)

Cobra (3 repetitions)
Locust (3 repetitions)
Bow (3 repetitions)
Spinal twist (1 minute to each side)
Yoga mudra (20 seconds)
Head-to-knee sitting (1 minute)
Tree (20 seconds to each side)

Pranayama (see Chapter 6)
Three sets of 15 repetitions of rapid breath followed by breath-holding; four repetitions of alternate nostril breathing.

Pratyahara (see Chapter 7)
Remain for 1 minute following the guided relaxation.

Concentration (select appropriate target)

Meditation (15 to 20 minutes)

Unification

This takes less than an hour. Add an additional 15 minute meditation period either morning or evening. You can break up the practices in different ways to fit your schedule. Each of the practices adds its own benefits; each builds on the effects of the last. Some people prefer to do the postures first and then meditate; others prefer to meditate before doing the postures. Regardless of order, each will benefit the other. I generally prefer to do the physical practices first to prepare for meditation. At other times, I will begin with a brief pratyahara relaxation followed by meditation. (See Appendix I for the 15 week somatic yoga program.)

6

Pranayama:
Breathing Exercises

The mind may also be calmed by expulsion and retention of the breath.

Patanjali

I have thoroughly enjoyed yoga and am really happy that I've learned it through this class. I have found myself remembering to practice it at stressful times (especially relaxing my breathing) and at times of intensity from which I need a break and need to relax and unwind (like during long periods of study). I find myself much less centered if I don't practice it and know it's because I need to take the time to relax and re-center. Before yoga, I didn't have any effective means of dealing with that uncentered feeling, whereas now I know practicing yoga is a perfect key. I have especially been practicing progressive relaxation, and have found it especially helpful as I'm often on a super high energy level, which I need to relax at times. If I don't practice yoga for a while, when I do it's like coming home again—coming back to myself, and it's so good to be there again.

Yoga student

In and out, exchanging oxygen and carbon dioxide, rhythmic and arhythmic breathing patterns in yoga practice are one more means of beginning to control your own inner core. How you are able to do this has something to do with stimulating the medulla located in the brainstem. Consciously changing the rhythm of your breathing is a little like taking the breathing into your own hands: the medulla, which is used to providing the rhythm automatically, is overridden by your imposed rhythm. By breathing deliberately, and mindfully, you are calling the shots yourself rather than in response to inherent rhythms and environmental events. This unusual process enables you to change the mixture of inhaled gases and the gaseous composition of your blood at will. Confused by this, the medulla sends messages up through the reticular activating system to inform the brain to be alert because something has changed. You maintain the unusual breathing pattern for only a brief time. This enables you to accomplish two things—to change the oxygen-carbon dioxide balance and tone up your organism.

Prana, considered the life force by yogis, is the primal energy from which all material objects evolve and to which all matter returns. The location of the vital energy in the human body is the solar plexus. It is believed that prana is stored there. Every form of energy comes from prana. All forces at the beginning of their cycles come from prana. At the end of their cycles they return to prana. When all forces in the universe—mental and physical—return to their original state, that is prana.

Pranayama is the training of breath control, a control of universal prana. The purposes for breathing exercises include psychophysical relaxation, rejuvenation, the release of dormant energies, and the creation of mental serenity. Psychophysical relaxation refers to the creation of a relaxation state through the alteration of the bodily state. Through breathing practices, this is achieved by increasing the oxygen content of the blood and clearing out lactic acid from the muscles by combining it with oxygen. The question of rejuvenation concerns the return to a more complete breathing pattern. As we get older, we tend to have increasingly restricted breathing. With the deliberate expansion of breathing capacity, we can in a sense return to youthful vitality. If you have ever heard stories about a little old woman who in a moment of crisis gained superhuman strength and lifted a car off someone who was trapped beneath, you have a sense of this release of dormant energies. Perhaps you have even experienced times in your life in which you have had an amazing amount of energy, far beyond your usual sense of what is possible for you.

Mental serenity is said to be achieved through equalization of the two breath currents. The left nostril (ida) and the right nostril (pingala) are considered to be female and male. These feminine and masculine currents—moon and sun, water and fire—are considered to be soothing, like water (moon), and electrifying, like fire (sun). The happy marriage of negative and positive vital (life) energies generates a new kind of energy. This new kind of energy is extremely subtle. It moves upward toward the seat of consciousness in the brain.

Mishra, in his book, *Fundamentals of Yoga*, discussed the physiological correlates of the breathing process and the neurological control of respiration. He mentions the cortical control over the medullary center, which is the location of the vital functions such as breathing, heart rate, and blood pressure. This breathing center is generally not under conscious control. The rhythm of that function fluctuates with the emotional tone and is controlled somewhat by the cortex's inhibitory mediating function. The other area from which breathing is controlled is the respiratory center in the medulla.

Mishra also mentions the cranial nerves involved in the breathing process. The cranial nerves—12 in number—are the peripheral branches coming from the central nervous system. The cranial nerves involved in the breathing include: CN V, trigeminal nerve; CN VI, abducens; CN VII, facial nerve; CN VIII, vestibular-cochlear; CN IX, glossopharyngeal; CN X, vagus nerve; CN XI, spinal accessory; CN XII, hypoglossal nerve.

Raja yoga does not emphasize external breathing practices. When you reach a certain state in meditation, you will automatically begin to practice a special internal breathing pattern. At one point you will, possibly, identify yourself with supreme consciousness. This is the perfect state of pranayama. Another state occurs when you forget movements of the chest during inspiration and expiration and identify with supreme consciousness. This is advanced pranayama.

Raja yoga breathing practices are done by will power only: you do not use your hands. In hatha yoga you may use fingers for alternate nostril breathing. Respiration can be voluntary or involuntary. You can alter your respiration pattern through cortical control, that is, through self-regulation. It is generally under reflex control. Respiration requires an integration of neuromuscular activity; there is also chemical or gaseous exchange. From the carbon dioxide tension level of the blood comes the information regarding breathing rate.

We will explore two kinds of yoga breathing patterns. One is rapid breath, or kapalabhati. The other is alternate nostril breathing. There are numerous other breathing patterns recommended by different yogis. These two will be quite beneficial to you.

Kapalabhati or rapid breath refers to abdominal or diaphragmatic breathing. Its purpose is to cleanse the respiratory system and nasal passage. It is said to stimulate every tissue of the body. You begin rapid breath from a comfortable cross-legged seated position, with hands comfortably cupped around your knees. Using the abdomen as your breath handle, pull the abdomen in as you exhale. Then inhale. Inhale and exhale as rapidly as you can. Breathe through your nose. Do not breathe too forcefully. Rapidly inhale and exhale about 15 times. Then take a normal breath and exhale. Breathe rapidly 15 more times. Take a normal breath. Finally take 15 rapid breaths. Complete the process by taking a breath and holding it. Keep your eyes open the entire time. Hold your breath as long as you can comfortably. Exhale. Breathe normally for a few seconds, being aware of the resulting sensations of your breathing practice.

As you take your breathing rate into your own hands for voluntary control, you will be stimulating the medulla. Your stimulation causes the medulla to send messages via the reticular activating system to various areas of the brain.

Alternate nostril breathing is an exercise in mindfulness. Every aspect of it is designed to capture your attention. Each time your attention wanders, you will notice that you have forgotten some aspect of the practice. Your attention will be brought back. Whereas in classical raja yoga you do not use your hands during pranayama, contemporary raja yoga or somatic yoga does use them during alternate nostril breathing. Using your right hand, place the thumb against your right nostril. Fold the index finger and second finger into the palm of your hand. You may wish, when you are beginning, to rest these two fingers on the forehead in the area of the third eye as a sort of pivot. With your right finger and little finger close the left nostril.

Now inhale through the right nostril with the left nostril closed by your fingers. Inhale for one unit or Om-1; close your right nostril (both nostrils are now closed) for four units or through to Om-4; open your left nostril and exhale for two units or through to Om-2. This will constitute one cycle.

Repeat the process beginning with the left side. Inhale through the left nostril for one count; hold your breath for four counts; exhale through the right nostril for two counts. Be sure your eyes are open. Breathe from the abdomen. Do not breathe forcefully enough to disturb a feather if it were placed in front of your nose. Perform this cycle once in the beginning. In subsequent sessions, you may wish to add repetitions up to 150. You will also want to extend the amount of time that you hold each step of the process. The ratio is 1:4:2. Change it when you are ready to 2:8:4. Inhale for two counts; hold your breath for eight counts; exhale for four counts. The upper limit of the ratio is 8:32:16. Do not push yourself. Extend the time when you are ready. One handy way of knowing when you are ready is when you lose count and find that you have gone beyond your present limit. If it is comfortable, you may feel ready to try the next level. Above all you do not want to panic, feeling out of breath. That would be a sympathetic nervous system stimulant.

You will find that pranayama practice as described above will greatly enhance your meditation.

7

Pratyahara:
Progressive Relaxation

Yoga for me this semester has meant getting in touch with my
entire body, mind and spirit. Since high school I have not used my
body very much physically. I was very out of shape and out of touch
with my own body, and my feeling for yoga this semester has been:
'get in touch with my body.' I feel I have accomplished this – I feel
very in tune with myself in every way – it has been a very beautiful
and centering thing for me. Being in tune with my body has made
me very in tune with my spirit – I feel centered, alive and full of
well-being! Enough so I am positive I will continue my yoga into the
summer and hopefully from now on. This class has been an inspiration and a fulfilling experience.

My body has really 'cleared' up, felt stronger, more balanced and
alive. And the same goes for my mind and spirit. It was a real positive experience for me as the *total* being.

Yoga student

Pratyahara means progressive body relaxation and sense
withdrawal. From this process of attention and withdrawal of
attention comes the ability to withdraw awareness from the
periphery of the body. Attention is withdrawn from the extremities and moved up through the body. Focused, concentrated, and
dissociated, it can now be centered in the area of the third eye, the
forehead. This enables us to put the maximum amount of attention, energy, and awareness into whatever we do. Greater
awareness – not inattentiveness – is the purpose of this practice of
sense withdrawal.

Evoked potential research indicates that a competing stimulus, resulting in division of attention between sensory systems,

causes a reduction of the response in the sensory mode not attended to. If you place your attention on a sensory mode, reducing the competing stimulation, and increasing the sensory input in that sensory mode, you will get maximum effects from the sensory input. Your undiluted response will be stronger.

Pranayama is active; pratyahara, passive. Pratyahara, when practiced repeatedly, has a cumulative effect and you become more effective in your relaxing and letting go of body tension. I do not use the progressive relaxation approach of Edmund Jacobson (1938) and Swami Satchidananda (1970), which requires the person to tense the muscles before relaxing them. Electromyographic recordings indicate that once the muscle contracts, once the muscle activity increases, it takes a while to relax again. The more a person tenses the muscle, the more it retains that tension. That kind of tension or contraction is difficult to release.

What's the alternative? I have the person place his attention on some part of the body; he suggests to himself that the area will relax. Then he pauses to feel the results of the suggestion: the perceived relaxation. I generally work with the large body areas; the mind is capable of orchestrating the specific activities required to relax the area. Repeat the suggestion three times slowly. Relaxation suggestions are, in general, very effective.

Here are the directions I usually give—one approach to pratyahara. For maximum relaxation you must give yourself permission to relax. Being alert and vigilant, responsible and self-directed, controlling and guiding, you need to give yourself explicit permission to relax. Lie on the floor with your feet about 20 inches apart and your hands palms up on the floor about 10 inches from your sides. Check your body to see whether you are holding on to any parts, to your pelvis, to your shoulders. Gently, wiggle your feet, your hands. Rolling your head on the floor is the last movement toward letting go.

Follow me. I will speak—quietly, in the first-person—because I am speaking for you and for me. When I mention each part of your body, place your attention on that area and suggest that it relax and feel it relaxing. Pratyahara requires the following steps:

(1) place your attention on the target; (2) suggest that it relax; (3) feel the effects of your suggestions.

Repeat to yourself: I am relaxing my feet; my feet are relaxing; I am relaxing my feet. I am relaxing my legs; I am relaxing my legs; I am relaxing my legs. (Do this with each area of your body: pelvis, abdomen, chest, back, hands, arms, shoulders, neck, head, internal organs, brain, face, jaw.) Finally, say: I am relaxing my entire body; my entire body is relaxing; I am relaxing my entire body and I am comfortable.

Deliberately relaxed, still awake, wholly still—remain in that state for approximately five minutes. If you can keep your mind clear, if you can maintain the physical relaxation, if you can sit up and retain that feeling of relaxation, then you will have achieved a state which is a great aid to meditation. You can even quickly repeat the process after you sit up to assure the continued relaxation.

Now that we have looked at the process of sense withdrawal or pratyahara, you are ready to begin concentration.

PART THREE

The Mind in Somatic Yoga

8

Concentrating the Mind

Concentration (dhrana) is holding the mind within a center of
spiritual consciousness in the body, or fixing it on some divine
form, either within the body or outside it.

Patanjali

It took me until the end of the semester to really get into meditation. At first I was bored and restless. Now I can stay with it the
whole time and get into a dreamlike state and come out of it
relaxed and sometimes with problems resolved.

Yoga student

Yoga includes a number of activities which facilitate concentration. Meditation, the degree of concentration permitting,
dawns in the conscious mind after extensive practice of concentration. Few are able to concentrate, fewer are able to meditate. The
more you concentrate, the more likely you will be to evolve into
meditation. That kind of evolution you cannot *make* happen. You
must use what is called "passive volition." You have to try without
trying. You have to allow it to happen.

Devoted to developing concentration skill, some procedures
use the eyes to fix attention; these are called tratakam or gaze
training practices. Some concentration exercises do not use any of
the senses, but only the mind. Some use the body posture; some
use no concentration target at all: meditation without seed. The
goal is to make the mind "one pointed." Concentration improves
with practice, along with your ability to function in many other
activities.

It is helpful if you set aside a room or portion of a room for your
meditation. If you do so you will find two benefits – you will begin

to associate the meditative state with it, and it is said that the area will begin to collect the vibrations from your practice. Of the two phenomena, we can at least recognize the environmental suggestion or conditioning effect. Quiet, natural, peaceful places for meditation are numerous if you become creative in recognizing them.

How you can remain in a fixed position for an extended period of time is something of a mystery. Remaining still requires a great deal of action on your part: the action is performed by inhibitory neurons or circuits within the neuromuscular system and related systems. Rising desires or thoughts or impulses to move are effectively blocked as they emerge.

The following categories are presented as possible meditation foci or targets. Students are encouraged to try various approaches; they are invited to choose the ones most congruent with their own natures. For every person there is a suitable approach to meditation, one that relates to that moment. Some approaches will come quite naturally, but not all of them. The meditation targets include: visual meditation targets, auditory meditation targets, tactile meditation targets, olfactory meditation targets, and gustatory meditation targets.

Visual Meditation

Providing the attention is focused on any object of your choice as a target for visual meditation and gaze training, any object can serve as your visual meditation target. The target—preferably, one of special significance to you—might be a candle (directions will come later); a mandala (classic or of your own design); the moon; parts of your own body; any person or another person's eyes; a blue light; your own inner lights; the picture of a liberated person (Indian guru or simply someone you admire); or your own mirror image.

With a visual concentration/meditation target, as with any sensory mode, you simply place your attention on the target and hold your attention on the target over a sustained period of time. This means that you must repeatedly return your attention to the target as your mind wanders. Therefore, it is useful to use some aid in holding your attention on the target. We use the Om-count. Count slowly from one to 10. Think Om on the inhalation and count on the exhalation. With each breath, return your attention to the target. If thoughts enter your mind, simply let them drift out again. If you lose your count, begin your count again.

Candle Meditation

Candle meditation is like meditation on other visual targets, but dissimilar in that a candle is an original light source. The state you achieve (your attention permitting) is one of calm, energized centeredness. The candle in meditation is a radiating light source; other objects are seen by reflected light. The candle—a flickering light—catches the attention.

To begin candle meditation, sit at arm's length away from it with the flame of the candle at eye level. Look at the candle flame for a minute; close your eyes and see the afterimage for a minute. Repeat this three times. Then rest your eyes for a few seconds with eyes closed.

Meditation on the Picture of a Liberated Person

Why you select a certain person or picture depends on a number of factors. Unconsciously admiring, you may not know precisely why you choose him or her. The reason you admire someone is based on latent qualities in yourself, and exists on a low level of awareness. It is said that absorption in the picture enables you to take on the qualities of the person on whom you meditate. Is this the awakening of latent capacities? Sometimes a guru will pass out a picture of himself. This is not due to vanity. He offers the picture as a meditation target or at least as an environmental reminder of the state of consciousness that he represents.

Inner Lights

During my meditative development, I began to see, with my eyes closed, a soft blue light. The inner blue light seemed to undulate fluidly at various rates, and even recede into space before me. Curious, I did not realize what it was until I ran across a reference to it in Ernest Wood's *Yoga Dictionary*. The fact that it has been experienced by meditators since ancient times validated my subjective experience. Is this a light on the path?

The blue light experience of meditation is similar to the experience of diffuse light which accompanied the surgical procedure developed by Wilder Penfield. In this procedure, patients received a local anesthetic, the skull and protective coverings were removed to expose the cortex, and the cortex was stimulated to determine exact localization of the epileptic foci. The patients reported a variety of experiences. From their subjective reports came the realization that stimulation of the occipital lobe yielded experience of diffuse lights, but not patterned lights. It is possible (future research permitting) that we will find that the internal lights of the meditators may result from internal stimulation of the occipital lobe.

Gaze Training

Tratakam is a yogic practice concerned with activities that train the visual gaze, the ability to fixate on a visual target. Few can achieve a fixed visual position, fewer can maintain that fixation for any length of time. From this practice comes the ability to steady your mind through limiting the sensory input to one input channel.

The nasal gazes are three positions of the eye. The nasal gaze accomplishes several things, including increased stimulation of the external eye muscles, relaxation of the inner eye muscles, and reduction of visual input. Doing the nasal gaze is a little like looking down when you feel emotional: it restricts the visual input, but also adds tension to the general mood. If you relax, if you place your attention on your nose and you hold that position for a period of time, you will stimulate the areas of the brain responsible for the position.

Mishra (1959) suggests that you will want to do both the nasal and frontal gazes. He does not mention *why* you will want to do both gazes. Mishra, authoritative and sometimes mysterious, presents many recommendations to be taken on faith. If you try them, you will discern the differences between practices and how their effects blend.

Auditory Meditation

An auditory meditation can use any sound as its target. Choosing a sound that is pleasing or meaningful to you, you will find it easier to relax and clear your mind. It is more difficult to remain attentive to the auditory target than to the visual target. The auditory target has a tendency to stimulate reverie. Your attention, a fluid awareness, can be placed on one sound, and, like a wandering child, can be brought gently back to the sound each time you notice it has wandered. It is helpful to use the Om-count as an aid to holding your attention on the sound, keeping your mind clear, and remaining relaxed.

Possible meditation targets include: the Om mantra; the nad sound at various levels; music, especially Indian sitar music; sounds of nature such as waterfalls, rain, surf; fountains; your own inner sounds; or your own personal mantra, self-selected or given to you by your guru.

Mantra Meditation

A mantra is a Sanscrit syllable, a vibratory sound which has an impact on the perceiver. How does it work? A language of ancient origin, Sanscrit embodies vibrations that evoke states in the speaker or listener. For every mantra there are four levels. The levels, which are subtle, vital, and significant, include, (1) the sound of it; (2) the meaning of the word; (3) the idea it embodies; and (4) the spirit (prana) of it.

Om is a sacred syllable. It is the universal vibration, the Absolute, the All; the human sound, a symbol representing the universal vibration. A sound or prolongation (nada), Om ends in a point which equals the material representation of the subtler universal energy. Omnipresent, omniscient, and omnipotent, Om is the statement made about the divine presence. Om is two things: the ground of meditation and the root of meditation or spiritual meaning—the "color" of meditation in the spectrum of the one sound.

An ocean of nad is flowing everywhere in nature. It is inside and outside of living and nonliving objects; everything depends on it, it is all powerful. It is omnipresent (everywhere present); it is omniscient (knows everything).

By listening carefully, you can hear the Om sound. You can hear it best through your right ear—it is a vibration without instruments. There are two ways to hear it. One artificial way is good initial training. It is a yoga mudra technique, translated roughly as "closing every hole in your head." If you close your ears with your thumbs, your eyes with your index fingers, your nostrils with your middle fingers, your mouth with your ring finger and little finger on the upper and lower lips, and breathe through your nose lightly, you will begin to see subtle, diffuse inner lights with Mishra says are the shape of your soul. You will hear mantra (a special sound)—anahata nadam—within your head.

The second method comes with practice. Not only will you be able to hear the nad sound by the above method, but you will begin to hear nadam without using the method. You will begin to be able to hear it anywhere as you remember to tune in on it, surround yourself with it, hear it within yourself. Anahata nada is said to be supreme consciousness manifesting through your sensory system.

Om has four states. The syllables of Om include "A," "U" and "M." The letter "A" represents "the manifestation and evolution of the microcosm and macrocosm" (Mishra, 1959, p. 201). "A" also represents the gross body and waking state. The preservation of the microcosm and macrocosm is represented by the letter "U." "U" represents the subtle body and dream state. The letter "M" represents "the dissolution and involution of the microcosm." "M" represents the causal body and the state of sound sleep, death and other unconscious states. The fourth phase is the echo.

From the vibration of Om comes a sound that is beyond human capacity for description.

The state of nadam is beyond the three states of Om—waking, dreaming, and sound sleep. It is a transcendental consciousness. It is called Brahman (the Greatest), and Atman (Self). It is the Absolute.

When you listen to the nad sound, you may hear the following sounds. First, a low roar. In the beginning you may hear the low roar, but not the higher sounds. From the low sound of your circulation comes a starting point which will enable you to find the higher sounds. You can find the higher sounds, which are subtle and quieter, higher and more vibrant, calm and peaceful, by listening toward the top of your head. These are sounds somewhat like white noise, wind in the leaves of the sounds of soft rain. When you can hear the nad sound inside, you will recognize it as similar to the above, but more subtle. The sound can serve as a guide: if you focus on it for a while, you will begin to hear a higher sound. What next? When you can hear the sound clearly, shift your attention to it, shift your level of awareness to that level. With the successively higher sounds your attention and consciousness is guided upward as on a staircase toward the transcendent, superconscious state.

There is one mantra which we do everyday: the breath mantra (sa ha). Natural, unobtrusive, and constant, it is repeated approximately 21,600 times per day. If we place our attention on it (our capacity to sustain awareness allowing), we are able to remain more aware of the "here-and-now," and to be relaxed and unified.

The mantra which suits your nature may have been given to you by your guru in initiation. The mantra may be a Sanscrit syllable, but it can also come from other languages as well. Filled with meaning, the syllable is also vibrational. The mantra, which has a stimulating effect on the auditory cortex, is either said, heard or thought. It is a focusing sound which serves to make your mind one-pointed and to synchronize brain rhythms.

Tactile Meditation

Tactile meditation—somatosensory, primitive, deeply satisfying—uses input through the sense of touch. An auditory meditation is difficult to sustain; a tactile meditation, even more so.

One form of tactile meditation, massage can be used in conjunction with yoga in several ways. First, there is the Esalen massage combination of massage and meditation which features an energy exchange between the masseuse and the person being massaged. Massage can preceed the yoga experience. The yoga practitioner can be massaged during various postures. Finally, the massage can be used meditatively, as with any tactile meditation. The massage, a benefit to both giver and receiver, can also be given meditatively.

Another form of tactile meditation is the use of prayer beads to help you count the repetitions of mantras or prayers. If you place your attention on the beads, turn them in rhythm with your repetitions of the mantra, and clear your mind, then after a sufficient length of time you will enter a state of relaxed, meditative awareness.

The telling of prayer beads is a sensorimotor experience which has an impact on brain function. When stimulation of an area of the brain is repeated for a sufficient length of time, the rhythm of activity spreads to adjacent areas. More and more of the brain begins to synchronize with the primary focus; a unique brain state can be achieved through specialized, repetitive input. Clearing the mind, attending to the sensorimotor activity, and facilitating the verbal repetition, each contribute to the effect of fingering the beads. Specific areas of the brain (competing stimuli permitting) are involved in each of these activities. If the beads were blessed by your guru, then you have additional confidence in the prayer bead practice, and a sense of its specialness.

Olfactory Meditation

Not only can you do an olfactory meditation, but the sense of smell can facilitate meditation. Because we habituate quickly to fragrance, it is difficult to sustain attention on olfactory input. To do an olfactory meditation, select any odor as a target, just as you would for any kind of meditation, and place your attention on it for a sustained period of time. A smell, an olfactory input, stimulates the olfactory bulbs attached to each hemisphere of the brain. The electrochemical impulse is transmitted via cranial nerve I to a primitive area of the brain—the rhinencephalon, part of the limbic system. Being ancient, primitive, and animal, the limbic system is very involved with our emotions and moods. Olfactory stimulation is deeply effective in aiding the meditative state through the use of incense, smells found in nature such as flowers, special perfumes and oils, and the special inner perfume which is said to accompany certain meditative states.

Gustatory Meditation

Taste can serve as a meditative focus as when a meal becomes a meditative experience. If we place our attention on what we are eating, clear our minds, relax, and perhaps repeat a mantra while eating, then it becomes a unifying experience and perhaps meditative. You can select a taste as a target: a flavor on which you can meditate, such as certain Indian candies which can remain in the mouth for a period of time.

Every Moment Meditation

From your personality type comes your orientation to life. If you are an intuitive type, you may find daily tasks are boring and tragically repetitious. For another personality type daily tasks are delightful, satisfying and fulfilling. Various approaches—games, exhortations, sheer determination—are only partially successful in getting yourself to perform daily tasks consistently. There is one gambit worth the effort. In this approach—every moment meditation—you attempt to transform every day into a meditative or attention training experience. If you perform a task and your mind is preoccupied with 10,000 other things, you do not effectively complete the task. Your body is present; your mind, elsewhere. You are not effective for two reasons—the task takes longer and the results may not be totally satisfactory. If you give full attention to the task by doing the Om-count or attending to your breathing while working, you will be able to complete the task more quickly and with greater satisfaction, a greater sense of closure. What else? There is also the benefit of converting distasteful moments in your life into positive contributions to your development. You can convert even irritating situations into developmental ones. Some situations can be and need to be changed; others can be used productively rather than wasting energy in fighting them. This is sometimes called "going with the Tao." The Tao is a term from Chinese Buddhism which can be used to refer to the balance of natural forces.

Seeing the World Freshly

Phenomenological perception is a kind of open perception or awareness in which we do not prejudge and label the experience. From earliest childhood we are encouraged to label the objects of our world. This process is very useful because it helps us categorize and differentiate, order our world, and make generalizations for further behavior. It also increasingly blocks us from valuable sensory input, from valuable fresh perceptions. Categorizing, standardizing our experiences, rounds the ends of sensations during the perceptual process and robs us of the excitement inherent in differences. This excitement is highly characteristic of childhood. Yoga training enables us to see the world again freshly, as children do. The concentration training practices of yoga are intimately involved with the development of refreshed perceptions. From the experience of concentration comes meditation.

9

Meditation:
The Communication Loop

Meditation (dhyana) is an unbroken flow of thought toward the
object of concentration.

Patanjali

The meditative exercise returned me to a much needed way to
self-awareness, self-sufficiency. I forget sometimes the powers that
exist.

Yoga student

My yoga and meditation act for me as a centering point in
which I live life. I meditate daily for an hour and have been doing
this practice for two years. I have been now doing hatha yoga steadily for one year. During the summer I am going to share what I have
been learning by teaching a yoga class in San Francisco. I am also
going to take a teacher's training course in Mexico with Indra Devi
which will certify me as an instructor. I feel that a lot can be gained
from yoga especially in the highly stressed society in which we live
today. Yoga helps me to travel through life in a flowing, calm and
collected way.

Yoga student

Meditation is elusive: it does not begin the minute you
try it. Concentration, contemplation—both are words which are
sometimes used to describe the meditation experience. Meditation proper is a state of consciousness—a state entered after a
period of time spent in concentration, relaxation, and stillness. If
you focus your attention, if you still your mind, if you remain
relaxed long enough, then your state of consciousness may
become that of meditation. Raja, transcendental, zen: there are as

many meditation styles or approaches as there are individuals who practice them. In hearing about these different approaches, remember one thing: they suit different personalities in different ways. Varied and similar, multicultural and interconnected historically, different meditation styles appeal to different people. If we use Jung's typology to differentiate different personalities, we would probably find a correlation between personality type and the style of meditation each chooses. You like the approach that suits you.

Whatever approach you choose, you will experience similar steps. Having placed your attention on your meditation target, and maintained it long enough, you will enter into the meditation state. This is a nonverbal dialogue between you and your meditation target. The instructions for meditation which Herbert Benson and others (1974) determined were cross-cultural, and include finding a quiet place, relaxing your body, and repeating something over and over for a period of time.

Somatic Meditation

The kind of meditation that I teach in my classes (I also encourage students to continue with the meditative approach that they already practice regularly) is an Om meditation. Taking a comfortable cross-legged position, which may be the lotus position or simply a cross-legged position, sit as erect as possible without overdoing it. You may want to put your hands in a mudra position with your thumb and index finger touching. The rest of your fingers comfortably extended, your hands rest on your knees with your arms straight (see Figure 9.1). Hold your head erect. You may want to place your visual attention on the floor about three feet in front of you — an angle even with the bottom of your nose. Or close your eyes: do a quick body scan with pratyahara suggesting that your body relax. Let each area of your body relax.

Now place your attention on your breathing. With each inhalation think Om and with each exhalation count from one to 10 consecutively. If you lose your count, start again. Breathe regu-

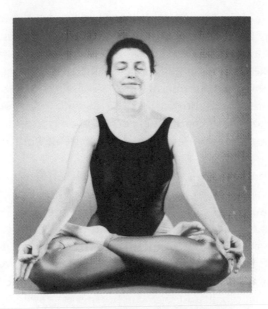

FIGURE 9.1a The Lotus Position

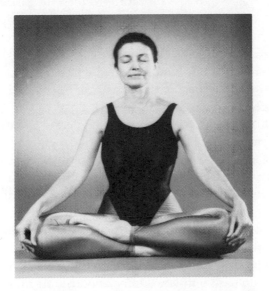

FIGURE 9.1b The Pose of the Adept

larly and comfortably. Om on the inhalation and count on the exhalation. With each breath, become more and more relaxed. Should thoughts come into your mind, let them go gently out again. Make a mental note that you will write down any important thoughts after the meditation is over if necessary. (Take a minute, after meditation, to record in your yoga journal any important ideas or insights that came to you during meditation. You may even want to evaluate the nature of your meditation session.)

It is important that you meditate for at least 20 minutes. If you only have five minutes, that will be helpful, but it takes approximately 20 minutes to achieve the relaxation response. Between 15 and 20 minutes you will feel a shift in awareness. This is reminiscent of the shift from the sympathetic nervous system dominance ("fight or flight" system) to the parasympathetic nervous system dominance. As you remember, the parasympathic nervous system is the rest, repair, and reproduction nervous system. With that shift there will be a variety of physiological changes. The changes include: decrease in blood pressure, increase in gastrointestinal activity (your stomach may growl, an index of appropriate changes), movement of brainwaves toward alpha, decrease in oxygen consumption, dilation of peripheral blood vessels, increase in the temperature of your hands, decrease in muscle tone, etc. All of these changes are part of the relaxation response that Benson and others have written about (Benson, Beary & Carol, 1974).

It is valuable to set aside a meditation period twice a day. It is a nice way to start the day; it is a nice way to end the day. Thus, your day is embraced by an experience of relaxation, calmness, and self-caring. In a busy schedule it is sometimes difficult to find an appropriate time. Finding a time for meditation is all the more important if you have a hectic schedule than if you have a schedule that lends itself more readily to meditation. Creativity is the answer here.

When you finish your meditation, it is important to ease your way gradually back into your daily activities. As you finish you may stretch and move slowly as you reconnect with the activities that you need to do. You may want to write a little in your yoga journal.

During your meditation experience, you may want to use visualizations or affirmations. Visualizations are mental pictures of desired experiences; affirmations are verbal statements about desired outcomes. With visualizations you may want to suggest various positive outcomes for yourself or others. These should be congruent with the flow of your life and life in general. Affirmations are positive suggestions that you give yourself mentally. They may be yogic suggestions such as Mishra's five great suggestions: (1) Thou are that; (2) I am Brahman; (3) This self is Brahman; (4) Consciousness is Brahman; (5) Eternal existence, consciousness, eternal peace is Brahman (Mishra, 1975). Or they may be ones that you design to fit your own needs. Mishra refers to these as post meditative suggestions. Whatever you select, it needs to be appropriate for your yogic development and your basic nature.

Reflecting on meditation in the light of physiological psychology you can observe the following phenomena:

1. You are repeatedly stimulating the area of the cortex with the input from your meditation target. For example, if it is a mantra you are repeating, it would involve Broca's area of the right or left cortex, depending on whether the syllable was meaningful to you or not. If you are using your asana as a meditation target, then the appropriate area of the sensorimotor cortex would be stimulated over and over. Ordinarily, we are used to changing stimulation repeatedly. In meditation there is an effort to continue to experience the sensory input freshly, to stimulate nearly the same area of the cortex over and over. In meditation, repetition is the spice of life.

2. You have blocked out as much competing stimulation as possible, i.e., your eyes are closed and you have chosen a quiet place.

3. You have restricted physical movement for a time; therefore, your have reduced the activation of the brain relating to movement.

4. You are quieting down extraneous thoughts to the extent that you can. Thoughts that do well up are not reacted to and allowed to subside.

5. You have inhibited the cortical activity which inhibits lower brain activities. The primitive areas of the brain (brainstem and lower mammalian brain) are allowed to function without the usual cortical inhibition.

I believe that these are the origins of the internal experiences of meditation. The internal experiences—seeing inner lights and hearing inner sounds (even tasting inner tastes or nectar, or smelling inner smells)—are probably the result of stimulation from the reticular activating system and diffuse thalamic activating system stimulating various areas of the cortex. This yields experiences similar to those elicited by Wilder Penfield during brain surgery. When he stimulated various areas of the cortex with electrodes, patients reported sensations such as diffuse lights or sounds. Thus, the meditator, whose cortex is quieter, is more available to the flow of electrochemical impulses from lower brain structures which may, from time to time, activate sensory areas.

Regardless of the physiological origin of these internal experiences, they nevertheless serve as valuable aids to meditative development. In meditation, what you are trying to do is train the mind to be able to remain focused for greater lengths of time than ordinarily possible. With that you need all the help you can get. For example, when you count in order to keep your mind on what you are doing, you will wake up at some point and realize that part of you has gone on counting and another part has begun to think about what is happening tomorrow. If you can focus your visual attention on an inner light, *and* count, you will notice again that you have continued to stay with the light and the count, but part of you is again off to other things. All of the inner experiences can help you hold your attention on what you are doing until it becomes effortless. Suddenly, you do not need to focus your attention deliberately. You are there. When you arrive at that place, your breathing may decrease in frequency. It is as if you do not need to breathe. You are very aware, but you are thinking of nothing. You are experiencing yourself as pure being.

Progress in meditation is much faster than you might believe. If you do your practice consistently, you will observe yourself traveling down a well-traveled path. You will read about meditative experiences in books and spontaneously recognize the experiences that you have had. This confirms that you are on the right track. To have someone—your yoga teacher or someone experienced in meditation—with whom to discuss your meditation experiences is frequently valuable.

The benefits of meditation have been widely communicated. There are changes in psychological states, such as a tendency toward decreased anxiety responses; there are changes in self-concept and self-esteem. You will feel better about yourself as a person. Some psychosomatic complaints, such as hypertension or muscle contraction headaches, may decrease. There are mood changes: you may notice yourself feeling happier and more loving toward others. You will be less irritable and more content with various aspects of your environment.

You do not have to do all of the yoga practices in order to benefit from meditation. Doing the physical practices is sometimes helpful in preparing your body for meditation. Some people do meditation to prepare for the postures; others do the postures to prepare for meditation.

Meditation Research

Before we look at meditation research, let's look briefly at what the electroencephalograph (EEG) measures. Discovered in 1929 by Hans Berger, a German psychiatrist, the EEG measures changes in electrical potential between two locations on the scalp. This is the electrical activity of the cortex, by and large, which radiates up through the various layers covering the brain, the skull and scalp. Sensors or electrodes are attached to the scalp. Electrical changes under the electrodes are measured by equipment in the form of comparison between the electrical potential of the two points on the scalp. This comparison yields wave forms which have been called brain waves. Brain waves—they are not waves in the usual sense of the word—are an index of the fluctuations in electrical activity of the brain. We have been able over the years to begin to associate certain states of awareness or consciousness with these waves.

The first wave frequency to be identified by Berger was the 8–12 Hz (cycles per second) frequency he called alpha. We have begun to associate that frequency with the relaxed waking state. The research done by Katsamatsu and Hirai (1972) on zen meditators reported in the literature began the popularization of the idea that alpha frequencies, meditation, and altered states of consciousness were related. There does seem to be a correlation between alpha and meditation. But not all alpha is meditative and not all meditation is alpha.

The other brain wave frequencies are: delta, 0–4 Hz; theta, 4–7 Hz; and beta, 13–30 Hz. Beta is the brain wave frequency associated with alertness and even nervousness. Theta, 4–7 Hz, has been associated with the burst of insight that accompanies creative problem-solving. Delta shows its greatest percentage during deep sleep.

Das and Gastaut (1955) found that their meditating subjects had increased alpha frequencies during meditation. There was also a decrease in amplitude (height of the wave). After meditation, there was a reappearance of the alpha rhythm with a decrease in frequency.

Katsamatsu and Hirai (1972) recorded the EEG patterns during zazen, sitting meditation of zen masters and pupils in Japan. One zen master began with beta activity in all channels. After a very short time in meditation, alpha waves were present under all leads. Eight minutes later the amplitude increased to 60–70 microvolts.

Katsamatsu and Hirai (1972) analyzed the kinds of alpha waves during zazen. He measured 18 experienced zen monks. These men also produced alpha waves.

Katsamatsu and Hirai (1972) described four states: (1) the appearance of alpha with eyes open; (2) a decrease in amplitude; (3) the decrease of alpha frequency; (4) the appearance of theta.

F. M. Brown, W. S. Stewart and J. T. Blodgett (1971) measured the EEGs of 11 subjects during meditation. Their EEGs were characterized by frontal 8–12 Hz throughout the 15 minute meditation period.

Schwartz (1973) compared a group of meditators with a matched control group. The meditators, relaxed, showed a higher eyes-open alpha during baseline recordings than did the controls. After the eight minute meditation, the meditators showed less eyes-open alpha than the controls. Schwartz hypothesized that was because visual stimulation is more intense following meditation.

Banquet (1973) followed this procedure. A baseline recording, five minutes with eyes open and five minutes eyes closed, was conducted for a meditation group and a control group. The meditation period was 30 minutes. With eyes closed, the control group relaxed for 30 minutes. Three minutes was used for coming out of relaxation/meditation—the transition period. Finally, five minutes of mental concentration on a thought or image completed the procedure. Then the eyes were opened. There were 12 subjects in each group; the meditation group had been meditating for an average of two years. The recordings were bilateral (frontal, central, parietal, and occipital).

The control group had a fluctuating alpha rhythm in four subjects. Eight subjects had a persistent alpha rhythm in the posterior channels. Most meditators, Banquet found, produced dominant alpha of 10 Hz (20 μV in amplitude). Toward the end of meditation there was an even greater abundance of alpha waves.

In the second stage of meditation, Banquet (1973) found alpha appearing only in short bursts of a few seconds duration. Alpha was found not only in the occipital and parietal channels, but also the frontal channels. What else did he find? He also found great correlation between both hemispheres with regard to frequency, amplitude, and wave form of alpha during some periods.

At the All-India Institute of Medical Sciences, Anand and others (1961) measured the EEGs of four yogis before and during samadhi, the unification state. The normal resting EEGs of the yogis showed dominant alpha; the state of samadhi was persistent alpha for all subjects. The amplitude of the occipital alpha increased to 50–100 μV.

Swami Kuvalayananda maintains that the EEGs of subjects practicing meditation showed reduction of alpha percent time and amplitude. That alpha was spread all over the head, but flattened.

Some meditators have been found to show theta bursts 5–20 minutes after the onset of meditation. Beta activity has been found in some regions of the scalp for some subjects. You might expect, as a rule of thumb, brain wave frequencies to be altered by the *kind* of experience the meditator is having.

Biofeedback Training and Somatic Yoga

What is biofeedback training? Biofeedback is the use of technological devices to mirror back to you the state of your physiology so that you may change that state in desired directions—toward relaxation, for example. If you have access to biofeedback instruments, they can be valuable aids to the practice of somatic yoga. Perhaps the center where you study yoga may have biofeedback equipment. Or a biofeedback center or practitioner may operate in your area. If you can combine your yoga practice with biofeedback training or use biofeedback monitoring periodically, you will be able to see objective measures of the results of your yoga training.

Some of the results you may expect from yoga practice include the following: an increase in skin resistance measured on the electrodermograph feedback device (measured in Ohms for resistance or micromhos for conductance); an increase in your capacity to increase alpha brain waves on both hemispheres; an increase in peripheral temperature as measured by the skin temperature feedback instrument; and a decrease in electromyograph (EMG) or muscle electrical activity. These are some of the common biofeedback devices that are available, and some of the physiological changes you might expect to see measured by them. As you are able to see tangible measures of your physiological state and your capacity to change it, you will become increasingly able to change it without instruments, and increasingly confident in your yoga practice. With increased confidence comes an increased capacity to do the practices effectively. This will increase your capacity to be fully aware, moment-by-moment, as you do your yoga practice. Ongoing mind-body integration is the goal of somatic yoga.

You can do any kind of yoga from the somatic perspective or add the somatic dimension to it. You can develop that kind of mind-body integration through studying somatic yoga or you may begin with one of the other yoga orientations and gradually add the somatic dimension. Meditation is the final step toward integration. The experience of integration, samadhi, is the subject of the next chapter.

10

Samadhi: The State of Union

Samadhi is unitive or identity consciousness. It is the experience of oneness or identity: it is the unitive experience.

In samadhi, the state of oneness, the mind becomes identified with the meditative target. It is a superconscious state in which the Absolute is experienced with total understanding and joy.

Haridas Chaudhuri

Yoga has meant feeling my 35 year old body grow younger and stronger. Feeling a desire for healthier foods. The end of drinking coffee. Being better able to step back from my children, allowing them to exist in their own right and me to exist for myself. Thoughts and attitudes and positive energy to send to a friend in prison. A chance to read several works on spirituality and synthesize these in a few instances. Discovering that Christianity, which I thought I had abandoned, was still a part of me and is the same religion for me as all other religions. Discovering I have a religion of my own based on seeking and loving God.

Yoga student

First you place your attention on your meditation target — concentration. If you are able to maintain the focus of your attention on your meditation target long enough — approximately 2½ minutes — you will cease to project meaning on your target. You will begin to receive information from your meditation target. Coming from the unique features of your meditation target, this information is a nonverbal communication. Thus, you have entered into a nonverbal dialogue with the object of your meditation, a communication loop.

If you are able to maintain the meditative loop long enough — approximately 28 minutes — you will enter into a state in which you cease to experience yourself as a separate self. You metaphorically or perhaps actually merge with the object of your meditation. This is samadhi or unification with the object of your meditation. This is the lower samadhi. Or what I call "little" samadhi.

In the larger sense, samadhi is the state of union with the Absolute. It is the ultimate goal of yoga—one that few of us will realize. Some people experience it for an instant. The goal is to be able to achieve samadhi permanently. A few Indian saints have been said to have achieved it. A few non-Indians seem to have achieved similar states.

There are little or lower samadhis and big samadhis. The little samadhis typically occur for a brief period of time, usually as a result of meditation. They can also occur during other activities. From the experience of ceasing to be aware of a separate self, you become ego-less. If the internal chatter ceases for a brief period of time, you experience yourself as being pure. It generally occurs when you are able to stay in the meditation loop long enough. For a period of time, you and the object of meditation become one. Whether this is a subjective experience, metaphorical, or actual on some plane of existence is not a final concern here. Just as there seems to be a unified field of consciousness, so too this seems to include the person and the object of his meditation.

At that point there is an experience of union. What is it like? This experience of union is somewhat like the big samadhi, the big samadhi which is a permanent union with the cosmic consciousness, God, the All, the Absolute. Some call it the ground of being. You may have another name for it. Whatever you call it, it is the ultimate goal of yoga.

There are two classes of samadhi (Mishra, 1959). The two classes are samprajnata samadhi and asamprajnata samadhi. Samprajnata samadhi would correspond to the little samadhi—fixation, suggestion, and sensation or dhrana, dhyana, and samadhi. It refers to enlightenment or the superconscious state of mind. "The body is fully magnetized, the senses go into the state of *yoganidra*, the mind enlightened, and the Self is awakened from its long sleep (ignorance)" (Mishra, 1959, p. 209). Body and mind unified, the body achieves a state in which it is able to tolerate the stresses of the ecstatic states. There is full development of eternal and divine intuition. The mind is fully focused on consciousness; it becomes enormously perceptive of internal and external reality. It is the state of union with the supreme consciousness. In this state — unified — you know the object of your meditation, not externally, but because you are one with it. The thought and object of thought are the same.

Asamprajnata samadhi refers to the transcendence of dualism. This is what is called nirvanam: it is one-without-a-second. There is no longer any separation between self and non-self, consciousness and unconsciousness. It is a very positive experience. When the mind enters this state, it does not return to the ordinary state of consciousness. There is no self and no non-self. It is a state that has been considered omnipotent, omniscient, omnipresent (all powerful, all knowing, and everywhere present). It is a state of eternal peace and happiness or bliss.

This state is not achieved by external practices. It is obtained by the power of the spirit alone. Mishra (1959) says that "every soul is potentially divine and has eternal existence, knowledge, and bliss in potential form" (Mishra, 1959, p. 219). That due to wanderings of our mind we have forgotten our true nature. That in the experience of asamprajnata samadhi this loss of knowledge is removed. Our infinite nature is revealed. The powerful omniscience, omnipresence, and omnipotence is returned.

The state of samadhi relates to humankind's evolutionary direction. It is said that there is a developmental process that occurs with each lifetime. Each lifetime contributes to the evolution of the person, each lifetime contributes to the next.

One aspect of yoga that has been highlighted repeatedly is the concept of self-realization. Sri Aurobindo felt that the ultimate goal of the person was self-realization (Chaudhuri, 1975). What is meant by this is both a realization of the unique self of the person and realizing the Self within. The latter is the recognition and identification of the Brahman within called the Atman. Yoga's concept of the evolved person fits very nicely with the notion found in the work of psychologists C. G. Jung, Abraham Maslow, and others.

The state of samadhi is very similar, if not identical, to the states of enlightenment mentioned in other mystical traditions. This is true of the Sufis; it is true of the zenists or the Christian mystics like St. Teresa. It is the state of evolved consciousness. Able to see the true nature of reality, the mystic follows principles reported by Evelyn Underhill (1961). She describes the situation as one in which the person experiences this ecstatic state and then returns to do service in the world.

It is important to recognize that this state of self-realization and enlightenment is a universal human aspiration. The world's religions and philosophies show that there are diverse ways and disciplines leading to this goal, but, nevertheless, it is still the same universal goal.

When the Sufi performs his ecstatic dancing songs to Allah, he is seeking Samadhi. When the Zen monk achieves an enlightenment that stays with him while doing the mundane tasks of fetching water and chopping wood, he has achieved Samadhi. When the consciousness of St. Francis emerges with his very soul and the soul of the world of nature, embracing all living creatures, this too is Samadhi. Samadhi, then, is not an exotic state peculiar only to yoga but is an achieved human state recognized universally.

The yogi, having had this experience on a small scale, can continue to live fully in society. Enlightened, it is then possible for him to live with material possessions and not be attached to them. Using the material world as a place to do one's dharma (life's work), you use the resources at hand. You are not bound by them; you have achieved liberation. It is a wonderful thing to be able to transcend the pains of existence just enough to be able to function more effectively in the world.

There are two dimensions for living: the horizontal and vertical dimensions. The horizontal dimension is the human-to-human relating on the material plane; it is full of emotion and suffering, love and joy. The vertical or transcendent dimension concerns humankind's awareness of existence beyond the personal dimension. When you are drawn to the vertical dimension, it is tempting to try to transcend the pain and suffering of life. With some measure of transcendence, you are released from the pain of existence. There is some measure of peace and calm. You find yourself missing something—you miss the fellowship of other humans. You miss feeling at the usual level of intensity. You cannot work as effectively with others because you cannot fully empathize with them. So you experience the situation which feels as if you choose to be a human being; you re-choose for the meantime in order to be able to do your work in the world. This choice relates to the householder period of your life. Later, when you have done the everyday kind of things, when your work in the world is done, you are free to experience the joys of the transcendent dimension more fully. You will feel content to move away somewhat from the intense emotions and pains of living as a human being.

In the meantime, a little samadhi will enable you to experience *this* world more fully. It will enable you to experience the state of oneness with objects, scenes from nature, persons you care about deeply. The experience of samadhi can enable you to expand your knowledge along lines which feel like the recovery of forgotten knowledge. The experience of samadhi can enable you to empathize more completely with others. It can enhance your feelings of love toward others, toward the world. It can enhance your perceptions in your daily life. It is said to free dormant energy within you. It will reduce your ego boundaries: your feeling of aloneness in the world will decrease. Your state of psychophysiological relaxation will increase.

We have no physiological research to validate the subjective experiences of those who have reported having the samadhi experience. To the outside observer, the individual *does* look altered. Ramakrishna was said to have glowed (Isherwood, 1970). If one has experienced the small samadhi, he may be able to communicate with us after the experience. If it is the larger experience, he is permanently altered. It is said that his contribution to the world becomes that of the effulgence of pure being. The experience of little samadhi is accessible to all of us with practice; big samadhi is precious and rare in human existence. This is as it should be; we have much to do before we leave.

> The Dew is on the lotus!—rise, Great Sun!
> And lift my leaf and mix me with the wave.
> the Sunrise comes!
> The Dewdrop slips into the shining Sea!
>
> *Edwin Arnold*

PART FOUR

The Psychophysiology of Yoga

11

The Psychophysiology of Yoga

Enchanted loom where millions of flashing shuttles weave a dissolving pattern, always a meaningful pattern though never an abiding one.

Sherrington

I have tried to integrate yoga practices into as much of my life as possible. I try to practice the postures every day both in the morning and evening and other times, too, but at first it came better to me in the evening. I really use meditation as a focusing and centering device – it really helps me stay clear. I say the Om count to myself throughout the day to help me relax and to help things to flow along more easily. For example, at work when things get a little hectic, the Om count and deep breathing help me stay calm and deal with the situation. I practice the Om count when I'm walking, riding my bike – these things can be like meditation to me. I also practice deep breathing at night. I have become more aware of my health, my breathing, my diet, my physical, mental and spiritual self.

Yoga student

This chapter is devoted to an exploration of the structure and function of the central and peripheral nervous systems. In somatic yoga it is important to understand how these systems work. Having a clear picture of how they work, you will be able to be aware of various functions as you do your yoga practice. This is the very essence of somatic yoga: the combination of yoga practice with the unification of sensory and sensorimotor awareness. The moment-by-moment awareness of the physiological effects of your practice is both the aim and the result of somatic yoga. For that reason it is valuable to read this chapter. As your read it, stop periodically and visualize how the structure might be organized within your own body. Mentally trace their functions. Then, as you do your yoga practice, bring into awareness again the functions stimulated by your practice. This approach will greatly enhance the results of your practice.

The central nervous system—the brain and spinal cord—receives messages and sends messages. As much as we may take this for granted, we must remember one thing: information coming in and out is essential for the well-being of our organism. These essential messages coming in and out are both neural and non-neural. "Neural" refers to the activities of the neurons. Neurons are the basic cells of the central (and peripheral) nervous system; neural messages travel by way of chains of neurons. From other directions come the non-neural messages which are humoral or chemical. The neural inputs to the brain come from the skin senses, eyes, ears, nose and visceral senses. The humoral inputs—plasma constituents and characteristics—include oxygen, carbon dioxide, glucose, temperature, etc. Your yoga practices are providing input to your brain.

If inputs to the brain are neural and humoral, then outputs are also neural and humoral. The neural outputs include messages to the glands (endocrine and exocrine), the smooth muscles, viscera (gut, sphincters), blood vessels, heart, skeletal muscles. The humoral output includes anterior pituitary messages to other glands. Stimulated by the various yoga practices, you are deliberately providing input to the brain. Neural and humoral information to the rest of the body will be the output from the brain stimulated by yoga.

Another area of brain research relevant to yoga is the exploration of right and left hemisphere differentiation of function. Individuals whose corpus callosum has been cut to protect the normal hemisphere from the spread of epileptic seizure activity have demonstrated some unusual abilities. In what way are they different? The person, although seemingly integrated, has two different personalities. The left hemisphere is responsible for speech. The majority of the population shares one trait in common—the trait of left hemisphere localization of speech. The left hemisphere is verbal; the right, non-verbal. The right hemisphere specializes in nonverbal abilities, but also abstract features. The right hemisphere, the left hemisphere permitting, is more holistic in its perceptions. There is a lateralization with regard to music – the right hemisphere is concerned with the melody. The right hemisphere – which is not simply mute, but also observant – is the central focus of yoga practices. From the facilitation of the right hemisphere comes a re-balancing of the two hemispheres. This re-balancing of the hemispheres leads to at least one thing: the synchrony of the hemispheres, an event which is seldom experienced in ordinary daily activities. By helping ease the dominance of one hemisphere over the other, this unification encourages greater flexibility.

We can also subdivide the cerebral cortex into lobes. The lobes, which are not really separate from the remainder of the cortex, make a convenient separation of functional areas. The frontal lobe has been considered to be involved with judgment and planning, experiencing a sense of self and responsibility. The temporal lobe has several functions, including dreaming and audition, and it is involved with remembering. The parietal lobe is concerned with mapping the body, blending the senses, knowing. Through yoga practice you are repeatedly stimulating certain areas of the cortex while quieting the activity of others.

Brain researchers have talked about the human as having three levels of brain. There is the reptilian level, which includes the brain stem upwards to the thalamus. Then there is the old brain, which we have in common with other animals – the limbic system. And finally, there is the neocortex or new brain. The function of the neocortex is primarily inhibitory with respect to the lower levels of the brain. In yoga practice, the task is to quiet the cortex. Its inhibitory function is eased. This allows the lower brain levels to function more freely. They can then contribute their homeostatic and motivational impulses to the organism.

The Neurons and Glial Cells

The central nervous system is composed of cells: the neurons and glial cells. The neurons conduct electrochemical impulses through the nervous system. How they are constructed is seen in the breakdown shown in Figure 11.1. Each neuron is composed of a cell body (or soma), dendrites which receive the information from other axons of other neurons, an axon which transmits the electrochemical messages to other neurons, and terminal buttons that are rounded swellings at the end of the axon. There are several kinds of neurons: multipolar, bipolar, and unipolar. When you provide sensory stimulation to the nervous system during your yoga practice, it will be conducted along the neurons by electrochemical impulses.

The other kind of cell in the nervous system is the glial cell, which supports, separates, insulates and metabolically sustains the neurons. Of the kinds of glial cells we include oligodendroglia, astrocytes, ependymal cells, and microglia. The astrocytes or astroglia surround the capillaries of the CNS forming part

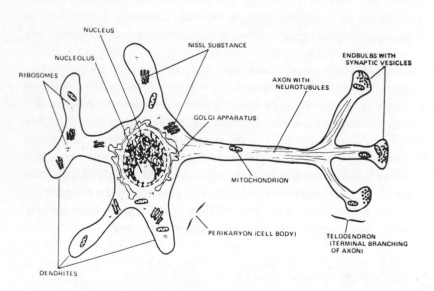

FIGURE 11.1 The neuron

of the blood-brain barrier. (The major part of the blood-brain barrier is formed by tight junctions between the endothelial cells which line the capillaries of the brain.) They permit certain sized molecules to pass from the capillaries to the nervous system cells, but not others. Engaging in numerous tasks, they transport metabolites, support and engage in housekeeping (clearing away the debris of dead cells). The microglia, the smallest glia, serve as phagocytes along with the astrocytes. The process of phagocytosis is the surrounding and digesting of dead cells and other debris in the nervous system. The oligodendroglia form the myelin in the central nervous system. The myelin sheath, a fatty substance produced by the oligodendroglia, helps insulate the myelinated axons. (Myelin isolates axons from one another; it allows for faster and more efficient electrical transmission.)

Messages are conducted along efferent pathways to the effectors of the body: the muscles and glands. Messages from the sensory receptors concerned with the muscles and glands return to the central nervous system; then help regulate its state. How are they used in somatic yoga? It is facilitating to the functions of somatic yoga to be aware of such activities – the messages being conducted along the afferent and efferent pathways – however subtle their signs may be.

When stimuli from the environment or within the organism impinge on sensory receptors, the ultimate effect is on the neuron. For example, a visual meditation target may stimulate the receptor cells of the visual system. If the input to a given neuron is sufficient to carry it beyond its threshold of excitation, it produces an action potential. The action potential is a brief electrical impulse that provides the basis for conduction of information along the axon: it represents brief changes in the membrane permeability to sodium and potassium. The neuron fires. When the action potential is produced it is propagated down the axon in an all-or-none-fashion. The all-or-none conduction is non-decremental and occurs in myelinated axons. Not only does it proceed in a saltatory ("jumping") conduction fashion, jumping from one node of Ranvier to the next, but also where there is no myelin sheath, there is a passive conduction of electric current. This passive or cable property conduction tends to decrease in strength as it progresses.

Neural Communication

The synapse is the junction between the terminal buttons at the ends of axonal branches of one cell and usually the somatic or dendritic membrane of another. Synaptic transmission is the way in which terminal buttons of axons send their messages across the synapse to the next neuron. Not only do they send their message across, but this message is transmitted only one way. Synaptic transmission is produced by the secretion of a transmitter substance produced in the terminal buttons. This transmitter substance is produced by the raw materials from the cell body of the neuron. This follows three clever steps: production of the transmitter substance, release of it, and deactivation of the transmitter substance. The latter is an important aspect of the cycle. If neural circuits get connected up at the synapses and remain connected, behavior will continue without change. So the transmitter substance packaged in synaptic vesicles goes through the following actions: migration to the presynaptic membrane, adherence, and rupture into the synaptic cleft. Then there is a recycling of the vesicular membrane. Finally, there is a termination of the postsynaptic potential through deactivation of the transmitter substance and re-uptake by the terminal button. All this is taking place as you do your yoga practice on an ongoing basis.

Postsynaptic potentials are the response of the receiving cells to the transmitter substance released by the terminal button of the transmitting cells. From this process comes integration by which inhibitory and excitatory postsynaptic potentials summate and control the rate of firing of a neuron. This is the process by which the neuron decides whether or not to send an action potential down its axon. As you provide physiological experiences through your yoga practice, you contribute to the postsynaptic potentials. In a complex way you are probably contributing to the preparatory state of your body by your sustained yoga practice.

Transmitter Substances

There are many transmitter substances. At least 40 or 50 have been identified (Garoutte, 1988). The transmitter substances have two general effects depending on the synapse: they are excitatory or inhibitory. The excitatory postsynaptic potentials (EPSP) cause a depolarization of the membrane. The inhibitory postsynaptic potentials (IPSP) cause a hyperpolarization of the membrane. The depolarization effect makes it more likely that the next neuron will fire; the hyperpolarization effect makes it less likely that the next neuron will fire. As you do your yoga practice, you will be creating excitatory and inhibitory postsynaptic potentials. In some parts of the brain, you will be contributing to excitation and in other parts, your effect will be neurologically inhibiting.

The most common neurotransmitters include acetylcholine, norepinephrine, dopamine, serotonin, and glutamic acid. Glutamic acid is the principal excitatory transmitter in the brain; GABA or gamma amino butyric acid appears to be inhibitory. Acetylcholine (ACh) is located at the neuromuscular junctions, the ganglia of the autonomic nervous system and at the postganglionic neurons which affect the target organs of the parasympathetic nervous system. Depending on the specific synapse, acetylcholine is sometimes an excitatory transmitter substance and at other times it acts as an inhibitory transmitter substance.

Norepinephrine (NE) has an inhibitory effect on neurons of the central nervous system. With target organs of the sympathetic nervous system, NE is excitatory. Dopamine (DA) appears to be inhibitory. For an inhibitory transmitter substance we have serotonin 5-HT or 5-hydroxytryptamine. Glutamic acid seems to be the principal excitatory transmitter in the brain. Appearing inhibitory, GABA is found in the gray matter and dorsal horn of the spinal cord. Glycine is an inhibitory neurotransmitter of the spinal cord and lower portions of the brain. Other suspected transmitters include taurine and aspartic acid and serine. They are amino acids concerned with excitation. Finally, there is a substance P, which seems to be involved with pain perception. We can infer from what is known about the secretion of neurotransmitter substances that your yoga practice is fully utilizing those mechanisms in complex patterns.

Chronic depression seems to be decreased activity in noradrenergic (and/or serotonergic) neurons. If there is increased noradrenergic activity, then manic activity is present. The calm that accompanies yoga practice points to the parasympathetic balance and the neurotransmitter substances, particularly acetylcholine, that are present in that state.

The Structure of the Nervous System

As you remember, the central nervous system is made up of the brain and spinal cord. The peripheral nervous system—the spinal nerves, peripheral ganglia, and the cranial nerves—include all nerves outside of the central nervous system. Yoga practices provide stimulation for both nervous systems.

The Brain

The brain is bathed in cerebrospinal fluid. Cerebrospinal fluid is a clear liquid somewhat like blood plasma. The fluid fills the ventricular system of the brain and spinal cord. It is a flotation system for the brain and spinal cord; it protects them. As you do strenuous yoga postures, your brain will be cushioned in its various positions relative to gravity by the CSF.

Blood supply to the brain is supplied by two major set of arteries—the vertebral arteries and the internal carotid arteries. The vertebral artery is an artery whose branches serve the posterior regions, the caudal region of the brain and spinal cord.

The internal carotid arteries serve the rostral portions of the brain. Strokes which cause aphasia are examples of difficulties with the internal carotid arteries: they serve the verbal areas of the left hemisphere or Broca's area. Recent research on changes in local blood flow and glucose absorption shows the effect of various activities on cortical areas. In the future, results from studies like these with regard to yoga practices should be highly informative for the confirmation of the somatic yoga approach.

Subdivisions of the Brain

The forebrain includes the telecephalon or "end brain." Three structures are located in that area – the cerebral cortex (Fig. 11.2), the basal ganglia (Fig. 11.3), and limbic system (Fig. 11.4). The basal ganglia and limbic system – subcortical areas – are located beneath the cortex. The forebrain also includes the "interbrain" or diencephalon; the diencephalon includes the brain structures called the thalamus and hypothalamus.

The outermost layer of the brain is the cerebral cortex. It is composed of neuron cell bodies, called gray matter because it lacks the white myelin sheathing that is around the axons of the neurons. The cerebral cortex is 20 square feet or so of cortical area covering the outer surface of the brain. If one looks at it closely, one sees the gyri (singular, gyrus) and fissures. The gyri are convolutions or folds of the cortex. The fissures are major grooves in the surface of the brain; the smaller grooves are called sulci (singular, sulcus).

We can divide the cerebral hemispheres into five lobes. Just as these lobes are distinctive, so too are they interconnected with the rest of the brain. These lobes include the frontal, parietal, temporal, occipital and limbic lobe. The limbic lobe is less obvious because it is located on the midsagittal surface of each hemisphere; it is also called the paleocortex. It is part of the limbic system which we will discuss later. The function of the cortex is primarily inhibitory. It enables you to stop unwanted behaviors, for example, so that the desired behaviors are available. Through yoga practice you are developing new inhibitory circuits for greater behavioral control.

The corpus callosum (Fig. 11.5) is the largest commissure or bridge in the brain. The corpus callosum connects the association areas of the cortex on each side of the brain. A fiber bundle, a commissure connects similar regions on each side of the brain. As you

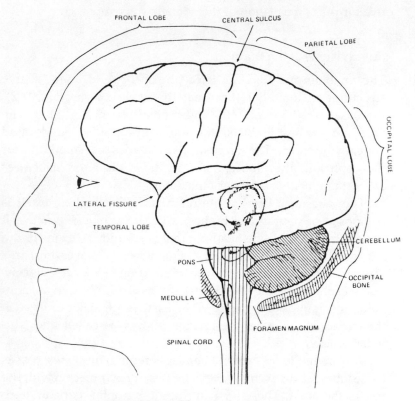

FIGURE 11.2 The cerebral cortex

do your yoga practices, you will be sending messages across the corpus callosum as you do bilateral movements, movements using both sides of the body.

The sensory areas of the cortex (Fig. 11.6) include the primary areas for sensory information: audition, vision, somatosenses (touch, pressure, temperature and taste) – all are included in the sensory areas. We will discuss how your concentration practices affect these areas of the cortex in Chapter 13.

The sensory cortex is a region of the cortex whose primary input is from one of the sensory systems. The motor cortex, located on the precentral gyrus, contains quite a number of motor

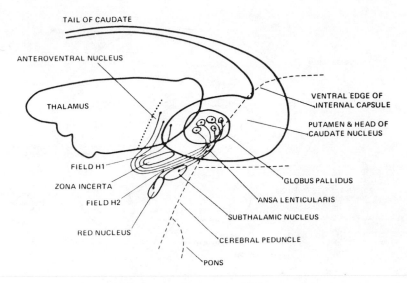

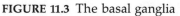

FIGURE 11.3 The basal ganglia

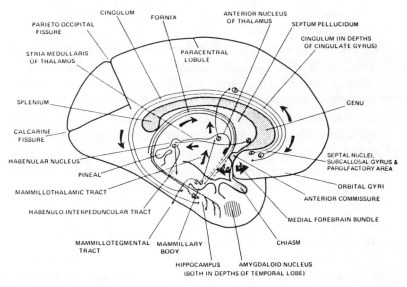

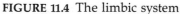

FIGURE 11.4 The limbic system

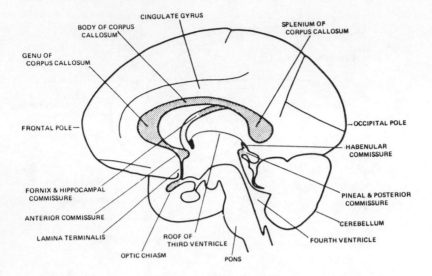

FIGURE 11.5 The corpus callosum

neurons. (See Chapter 12 for the effect of yoga practice on the sensorimotor cortex.)

Broca's speech area is a region of the frontal cortex. It is located at the base of the left precentral gyrus. It is necessary for speech production. The association areas are concerned with bringing together the sensory input to produce meaning. You would be using this area in chanting and mantra repetition.

The limbic system (Fig. 11.4) is a group of brain structures including the anterior thalamus, amygdala, hippocampus, limbic cortex and parts of the hypothalamus. It also includes thin interconnecting fiber bundles which connect the structures. The limbic system is involved with emotional and motivational behavior. It may also be involved with memory.

The hippocampus is a structure located in the forebrain portion of the temporal lobe. It has been implicated in two functions—learning and memory.

The amygdaloid complex or amygdala is a set of nuclei located at the base of the temporal lobe. The amygdala—"almond"—has

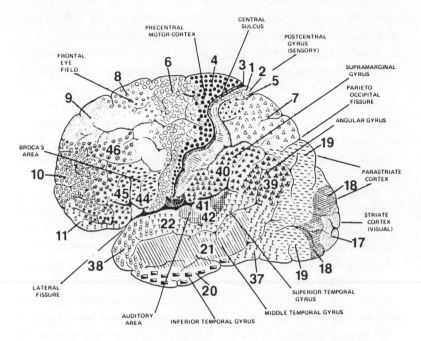

FIGURE 11.6 Sensory areas of the cortex (after Brodmann)
(Garoutte, 1987, p. 144)

been implicated in aggression. The septum or septal region is part of the limbic system located between the walls of the anterior portions of the lateral ventricles. The septum has been implicated in the control of the amygdala. It helps reduce aggressive behaviors.

The anterior thalamus is actually three thalamic nuclei, which receive fibers from the mammillary bodies. They project fibers to the cingulate gyrus.

The mammillary body protrudes from the bottom of the brain. It is located at the posterior end of the hypothalamus, and contains the medial and lateral mammillary nuclei.

How does your yoga practice affect the limbic system? You will notice the effect of your yoga practice on your limbic system indirectly. You may notice changes in your emotional state: increased calmness, decreased worry, or pleasant emotions. You may notice changes in motivations such as changes in eating behaviors or work habits. Learning or memory may seem to be enhanced. All are possible indications of limbic system involvement.

The basal ganglia (Fig. 11.3) are concerned with motor control. They are also concerned with emotion. Including the amygdala, globus pallidus, and neostriatum (caudate nucleus and putamen), the basal ganglia is concerned with various aspects of movement. Your yoga practice will utilize parts of the basal ganglia in various ways. For example, the caudate nucleus is involved with stopping movement. As you take and hold a yoga posture, you are probably involving your caudate nucleus.

The thalamus has two lobes connected by the massa intermedia. How is it constructed? The neurons with their cell bodies in the thalamus project to various areas of the brain. Axons of the neurons, these projections are efferent connections between neurons in one area of the brain to neurons in another area. From cell bodies located in one region of the brain, projection fibers are sets of axons. They synapse on other neurons located within another specific region of the brain. The information you send to your CNS from your yoga practice will synapse first on relevant nuclei of the thalamus before going on to the area of the cortex with which it is connected.

The hypothalamus (Fig. 11.7) is involved with five functions. The functions of the hypothalamus are categorized into five general types: (a) control of water intake and excretion; (b) control of temperature of the body; (c) control of reproductive functions, including secondary sex characteristics; (d) control of food ingestion, assimilation and appetite; and (e) control of daily rhythms ("circadian") (Garoutte, 1988). The hypothalamus—highly important for homeostasis—controls the autonomic nervous system. It is concerned with reflex integration. Not only does it control the endocrine system, but it is also concerned with the organization of behaviors related to survival of the species. The pituitary stalk attaches the pituitary gland to the hypothalamus.

The second major division of the brain, just below the diencephalon, is the mesencephalon or midbrain. It includes the brain

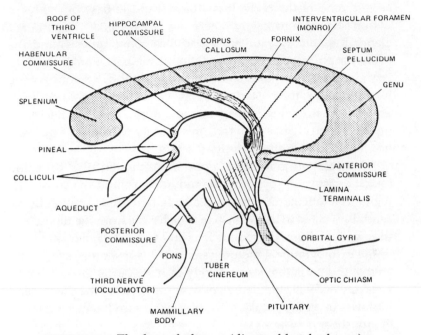

FIGURE 11.7 The hypothalamus (diagonal hatched area)

structures referred to as the tectum ("roof") and tegmentum ("floor"). The tectum is made up of the inferior and superior colliculi. The tegmentum is the portion of the midbrain below the tectum. It contains the red nucleus and nuclei of various cranial nerves. Some of the visual exercises and similar practices in yoga using other senses provide stimulation to the superior and inferior colliculi.

The tectum structures include the superior and inferior colliculi. From the old term corpora quadrigemina, "body of four twins," we see that there are four bulges. The superior colliculi are protrusions of the midbrain. They are part of our visual system, part of the residual primitive visual area. The inferior colliculi are protrusions of the midbrain also. They relay auditory information to the medial geniculate nucleus.

The pituitary gland has been considered the "master endocrine" gland of the body. It is attached to the base of the brain within is own bony cavity. There are two areas of the pituitary gland: the anterior pituitary gland (adenohypophysis) and the posterior pituitary gland (neurohypophysis). The anterior pituitary gland secretes hormones in response to the hormones of the hypothalamus, the posterior pituitary gland secretes oxytocin or antidiuretic hormone in response to stimulation from its neural input. As you change hypothalamic activity with your yoga practice, you will also affect pituitary activity.

The tegmentum includes a portion of the reticular formation (reticular activating system), the red nucleus, and the substantia nigra. The reticular formation is a large network of neural tissue centrally located in the brainstem which runs from the medulla to the diencephalon. The red nucleus and substantia nigra are parts of the extrapyramidal motor system. The substantia nigra is the area of the pons that stains darkly in histological analysis. Your yoga practice will stimulate all of your senses and, therefore, send impulses up your reticular activating system to change your levels of arousal and awareness.

The third major division of the brain is the hindbrain. The hindbrain is further divided into the metencephalon and myelencephalon. The metencephalon includes the brain structures called the cerebellum and pons. The myelencephalon, the most caudal division of the brain, is made up mainly of medulla oblongata.

The cerebellum or "little brain" is like a miniature replica of the cerebellum. How is it similar? It has a cerebellar cortex or outer layer. Its deep cerebellar nuclei project to the cerebellar cortex; cerebellar peduncles connect it to the rest of the brain. The cerebellar peduncles (superior, middle, inferior) are bundles of white matter. They connect the cerebellum to the brain stem. All of your smooth yoga movements will involve the cerebellum.

The pons is a region of the brain rostral to the medulla and caudal to the midbrain. The most caudal region, the myelencephalon includes the reticular activating system and nuclei. It also includes the medulla oblongata or medulla. The functions of the medulla include regulation of the cardiovascular system, respiration, skeletal muscle tonus and several cranial nerve nuclei. These functions are all altered by yoga practices and, therefore, involve the medulla.

Having discussed the impact of yoga practices on the central nervous system, we will now explore the peripheral nervous system's involvement with yoga in the next chapter.

12

Asanas: How They Work

Posture (asana) is to be seated in a position which is firm but relaxed.

Patanjali

Yoga has been extremely beneficial in helping me to recontact and communicate with my body. I am sure that what I have learned in this class will remain with me for the rest of my life. I am looking for a quiet space where I can practice yoga daily.

I have had dreams relating to this class, and this morning before class I dreamed that I held hands with the instructor and thanked her for all that she taught us.

Yoga student

The asanas or postures (static exercises) are a series of body positions designed to be held for several seconds or minutes. What is their purpose? The postures which are poised, quiet, and graceful are designed to stimulate various areas of the brain and body. This chapter will look at how the asanas affect the sensorimotor and related systems. This information is necessary for the complete practice of somatic yoga.

The postures (many of them are named after animals or objects) also serve as attitudinal reminders. The postures have three basic effects: relaxation, revitalization, and harmonization of body systems. They are an aid to meditation and bodily fitness. In hatha yoga, the physical practice is the goal; in raja yoga the postures are used as meditative experiences or are preparatory to meditation. That kind of differentiation is irrelevant in the end; it is said that both approaches lead to the same place. Having taken the variety of practices to the limit, the result is the same: union.

We have discussed the basic postures in Chapter 5; let's look at what is happening in your body when you do them. It will enable you to remain aware of your body's processes as you do the postures. Therefore, we will take time to look at how the spinal cord, spinal nerves, and the sensorimotor system are constructed (structure); we will also look at how they work (function). To get maximum benefit from this information, follow the steps below:

1. Read the text, then look at the picture or figure;

2. Gaze at each picture for 10 seconds;

3. Close your eyes for 10 seconds. See the picture in your mind's eye;

4. Imagine that structure in some part of your body (the muscles of your arm, for example);

5. Imagine this function occurring as you actually move your arm.

You do not need to be too precise in your exploration of this exercise. Just get a sense of it. Your soma will take care of the rest. Later, you will use this same process while you are doing the postures.

The Spinal Cord (Figure 12.1)

The spinal cord is part of the central nervous system as was discussed in Chapter 11. The spinal cord is composed of ascending and descending axons and cell bodies of neurons. The 24 individual vertebrae of the vertebral column protect the spinal cord. The function of the spinal cord is to serve as a pathway for fibers to the effectors of the body (glands and muscles); it also receives somatosensory information to be returned to the brain. As you do your yoga practices you are sending messages up and down your spinal cord.

There are 8 cervical nerves, 12 thoracic nerves, 5 lumbar, 5 sacral and 1 coccygeal. The sacral and coccygeal are fused vertebrae forming a solid structure. The spinal roots are bundles of axons. Surrounded by connective tissue, the spinal roots occur in

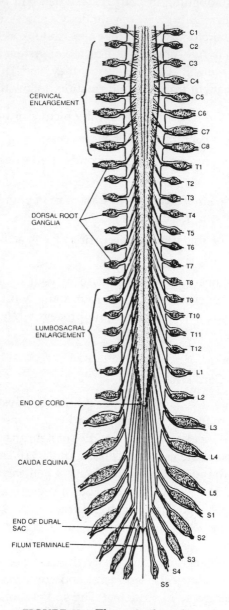

FIGURE 12.1 The spinal cord

pairs and fuse to form a spinal nerve. Extending beyond the spinal cord and to the lower extremities, the cauda equina or "mare's tale" is made up of spinal nerves. The dorsal root of the spinal cord contains afferent fibers: these are sensory. The ventral roots contain efferent fibers; they deal with motor function. The spinal nerves send information about your yoga practices to and from your spinal cord and brain.

The intercostal nerves are paralleled by the intercostal arteries and veins. There are nerve plexuses—a plexus (braids) is a network of several nerves—at various levels of the body. The spinal nerves fuse together and then divide again. The nerve plexuses have been associated with the chakras of yoga.

Muscles

Mammals (including humans, of course) have three types of muscles. Not only do they have the skeletal muscles (striated with bands and stripes), but also smooth muscles (lacking striations) and cardiac muscle. Yoga practice affects all three kinds of muscles, as we will see later.

There are two types of smooth muscles and they function automatically: they are the multi-unit smooth muscles and the single-unit smooth muscles. The multi-unit smooth muscles are found in larger arteries, around hair follicles and in the eye (affecting lens adjustment and pupillary dilation), but not elsewhere. These muscles are normally inactive—they respond only to neural stimulation or certain hormones. These muscles are the ones that contract when the sympathetic nervous system reacts to stress. Yoga practice enables you to decrease sympathetic nervous system outflow to these muscles. This decrease in sympathetic nervous system activity enables you to increase blood flow to the periphery of your body, and move toward relaxation.

Cardiac muscle looks like striated muscle. Pulsing automatically and rhythmically, it acts like a single-unit smooth muscle. Heart rate is modulated by neural impulses and certain hormones. There is a functional pacemaker: this is made up of a group of cells. If it is innervated, if it is given proper nutrition, if it has sufficient oxygen, then it rhythmically contracts the heart muscle. Yoga practice has been shown to slow heart rate and stabilize it.

Skeletal muscles are attached to bones. From that position they are able to cause bones to move relative to one another. Long and fibrous, striated muscles extend from their origins to their insertions. There are some exceptions. How are they connected? Tendons — strong bands of connective tissue — attach the muscles to the bones.

There are two types of skeletal muscles: flexors and extensors. Both types have only one function, that of contracting: contracting when the limb moves away from the body, contracting when it returns. The flexor muscles, ventrally located, bring the limb in toward the body when they contract. The extensor muscles have one effect: moving the limb away from the body. The extensor muscles are the antigravity muscles. Reacting to the pull of gravity, they help us stand up.

Yoga practice affects all three kinds of muscles. The more you do your yoga practice, the more you will affect the smooth muscles. Your degree of practice permitting, you will move toward a greater parasympathetic nervous system balance. These practices include meditation, pratyahara, and pranayama. The yoga practices which affect cardiac muscle are similar. Both kinds of smooth muscles are affected by changes in the autonomic nervous system.

Of particular importance is the effect of yoga on the skeletal muscles or the somatic nervous system. The asanas stimulate contractions of the skeletal muscles — the flexors and extensors. Let's look at the anatomy of the skeletal muscles.

Anatomy of the Skeletal Muscle

There are two types of muscle fibers: extrafusal and intrafusal muscle fibers. The extrafusal muscle fibers contract, providing the force exerted by the muscle.

Small and arranged in parallel with the extrafusal muscle fibers are the intrafusal muscle fibers. Functioning as stretch receptors, they detect muscle length. An afferent nerve ending is connected to `the capsule of the intrafusal muscle fiber. The intrafusal muscle fibers are found within muscle spindles. The muscle spindles are mechanoreceptors: they respond to forces applied to the ends of the intrafusal muscle fiber. As you do your yoga postures you will be stretching various muscles, stimulating mechanoreceptors.

The motor unit includes a lower motor neuron and its related muscle fibers. If we trace its path, if we consider its functional relationship, then we will include the alpha motor neuron with its axon and related extrafusal muscle fibers in the motor unit. It is a functional unit. As you do your asanas, you will stimulate various motor units causing contraction of all their muscle fibers.

The Neuromuscular Junctions

The neuromuscular junction is the synapse between the terminal buttons of an axon and the muscle fiber. On the surface of the muscle fibers is a specialized region, the motor end plate. The synapse of the efferent axon is the area where the terminal buttons meet the muscle fiber. The end plate potential is caused when an axon fires; acetylcholine is released by the terminal buttons. A depolarization of the postsynaptic membrane—called the end plate potential (EPP)—is caused by the acetylcholine. It is larger in magnitude than the similar excitatory postsynaptic potential (EPSP) in the CNS. It is important to remember one thing: the EPP always causes a healthy muscle fiber to contract.

The lower motor neuron is found in three locations: the intermediate horn, the ventral horn of the gray matter of the spinal cord, and in one of the motor nuclei of the cranial nerves. Its axon then synapses on the muscle fibers upon which it impinges. As you do your yoga postures, you will be sending impulses along the lower motor neuron to cause the secretion of acetylcholine from the terminal buttons and the end plate potential.

Muscle Contraction

The average rate of firing of the various motor units determines the strength of muscle contraction. Stretch receptors—muscle spindles and sensory endings—are sensitive to stretch of the muscle (Figure 12.2). They are arranged parallel to the extrafusal muscle fibers. The stretch receptors are activated by one signal: when the muscle lengthens. Therefore, they also serve as muscle length detectors.

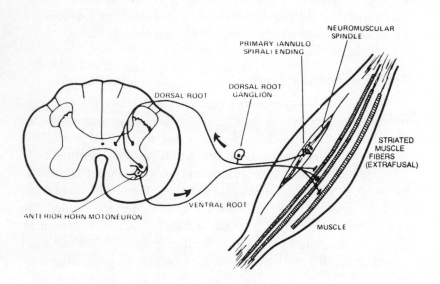

FIGURE 12.2 The stretch receptor

The Golgi tendon organs are located at the junction of the tendon and muscle. They hold stretch receptors, are sensitive to stretch, and encode the degree of stretch by rate of firing—all are aspects of the Golgi tendon organs' function. They are a prime target for yoga.

Stretch Reflex Systems

There are two stretch reflex systems: the monosynaptic stretch reflex and the polysynaptic reflex pathways. The monosynaptic stretch reflex has essentially one synapse; it brings the limb back to its original position. It is quick, simple, and involuntary. An example of this reflex is the patellar reflex. Remember all those medical examinations when the doctor tapped you just below the knee? A reflex is a simple circuit: it is defined as a motor impulse that is reflected back to the muscle. The monosynaptic stretch reflex (prevalent in yoga) begins with the sensory endings of the intrafusal muscle fiber, its afferent fiber. It synapses on its extrafusal muscle fibers in the same muscle. When the muscle is quickly stretched, then this reflex causes it to contract. An example is the gastrocnemius or large muscle in the calf. From the contractions of this muscle comes our ability to remain in a standing position. The reflexes that help maintain balance are very essential in yoga practice.

The Polysynaptic Reflex Pathways

There are many kinds of polysynaptic reflexes. Polysynaptic reflex pathways have many synapses. When there are a number of axonal branches, we have a divergence of information. When we have multiple input on a single neuron, we have a convergence of information. Complex and multi-synaptic, the job of the polysynaptic pathway originating from the Golgi tendon organ, for example, is to decrease the strength of muscular contraction.

Muscles are arranged in opposing pairs. Called the agonist and antagonist, they work against one another. The agonist moves the limb. The antagonist moves the limb back in the opposite direction. Not only does the stretch reflex excite the agonist, but it also inhibits the antagonist. As you do your yoga postures, you will be contracting various opposing pairs of muscles, various agonists and antagonists. You might take time to be aware of which muscles are contracting as you do various postures.

The Gamma Motor System

Muscle spindles are sensitive to changes in the length of the muscle (Figure 12.3). As the brain determines the length of the muscle spindles, it determines the length of the entire muscle. How is this done? The brain establishes a rate of firing of the gamma motor neuron (Figure 12.4). The gamma motor neurons are nerve cells sending efferent axons to the muscle spindles. Their sensitivity is adjusted by changing the rate of firing of the associated efferent fibers.

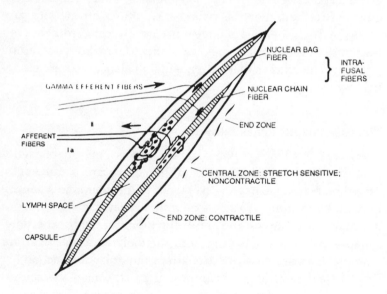

FIGURE 12.3 The muscle spindle

There is no muscular activity present while the muscle is resting. "Muscle tone," a non-specific term, depends on the gamma motor neurons. Gamma motor neurons—an auxiliary system—send impulses to the muscle spindles. The rate of firing of the gamma motor neurons is subtle, involuntary and it determines

the degree of muscle tone. As you practice the relaxing yoga postures and other practices, you will be able to regulate the activity
of the gamma motor neurons and muscle tone.

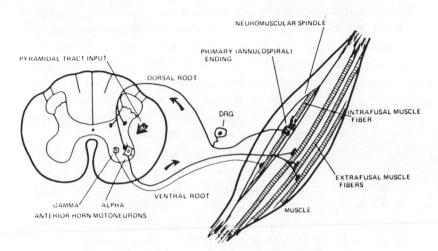

FIGURE 12.4 The gamma motor neuron

The Pyramidal Motor System

The "association" areas of the cortex participate in the initiation of
movement. Damage to this system causes altered movement,
often a robot-like movement. The pyramidal tract has to do with
the force of movement rather than the extent of movement. The
reticulospinal fibers make up the pathway which includes the
reticular activating system and the spinal cord. Portions of the
reticular activating system permitting, this pathway plays a role in
the control of the gamma motor system. The pyramidal system, a
crossed system, is involved with cutaneous pressure and the
maintenance of posture. The pyramidal system is responsible for
producing movement. The somatosensory input is the only *direct
input* to the motor cortex. The other input comes by way of the
multi-synaptic pathways. The decision to do a yoga posture
would involve the participation of the pyramidal motor system.

The Extrapyramidal Motor System

Whereas the pyramidal system produces movements, the extrapyramidal system smooths out movement. The extrapyramidal system has another function: postural adjustment to support these movements. What is its structure? That it is more complicated than the pyramidal system is clear. The extrapyramidal — "other than pyramidal"—has many synapses and is diffuse. It includes the neostriatum ("new grooved structure"), the caudate nucleus and the putamen. The paleostriatum ("old groove structure"), the globus pallidus, are also included. Yoga postures particularly utilize the extrapyramidal motor system.

The basal ganglia facilitates and inhibits motor sequences. The globus pallidus facilitates movement. If we look at what happens when any of these structures is disrupted, we can see their role in movement behavior. For example, the patient's ability to perform slow, smooth movements is interfered with by damage to the basal ganglia. Damage to the caudate nucleus or putamen results in major deficits such as rigidity or "uncontrollable writhing movement." If there is damage to the globus pallidus or ventral thalamus, then there is major movement deficiency or akinesia.

The cerebellum has three functions (Figure 12.5 & Figure 12.6). From research on cerebellar function we see that it receives kinesthetic and vestibular input. With that information it interacts with the brainstem, reticular formation or reticular activating system (RAS): the RAS affects the gamma motor system. Not only does it receive vestibular information, but it also exerts control over the postural muscles. This control is transmitted over cerebrovestibulspinal pathways. The neocerebellum is the latest developmental layer of the cerebellum; it is involved in the production of rapid, skilled movements. The cerebellum receives information from yoga activities; it sends out information to facilitate the movements.

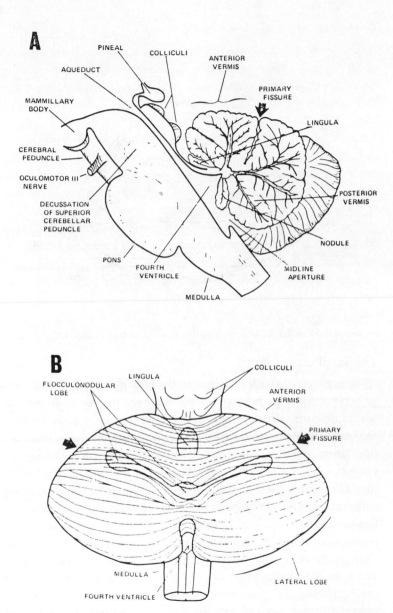

FIGURE 12.5 The cerebellum

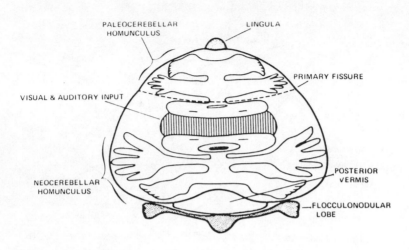

FIGURE 12.6 The localization of the cerebellum

The Vestibular System

In doing yoga postures, your body will be aligned relative to gravity in different positions. Moving into the postures will also stimulate your vestibular system. The vestibular system includes the bony labyrinths. The bony labyrinths enclose three structures (the "membraneous labyrinth"): the vestibular sacs, the semicircular canals, and the cochlea. If we look at the stimuli for the vestibular system, we must look at their effect on the two components of the vestibular system: the semi-circular canals and the vestibular sacs. The semi-circular canals respond to angular acceleration—the acceleration present in rotation. Detecting changes in rotation of the head, they do not detect steady rotation. There are three major planes of the head in which these canals reside: the sagittal, transverse, and horizontal. The vestibular sacs respond to the force of gravity. They inform you of your head's orientation in space, not your body's.

Kinesthesia and Organ Sensitivity

Kinesthesia refers to the sensory feedback from the movement and position of your limbs. Organic sensitivity refers to feelings from your internal organs. The kinesthetic stimuli come from stretch receptors located in two places: stretch receptors in the muscles indicate change in muscle length, stretch receptors in the tendons indicate the force being exerted by muscles. The intrafusal muscle fiber is a muscle fiber that functions as a stretch receptor. The fibers are arranged parallel to the extrafusal muscle fibers: they are muscle length detectors. As you do your yoga postures, you will be repeatedly receiving kinesthetic feedback.

The Golgi tendon organ, a receptive organ, is located at the junction of the tendon and muscle. It is sensitive to stretch. The fascia, a sheet of fibrous connective tissue, encases the muscle.

Kinesthetic and organic information is transduced by mechanoreceptors and pain receptors. They are like the receptors in the skin. The route of the kinesthetic and organic afferent fibers to the CNS shows that painful stimuli from the kinesthetic and organic receptors accompany sympathetic fibers; non-painful sensations accompany nerves containing parasympathetic afferents. You will be repeatedly sending impulses along the kinesthetic afferents as you do your postures.

There are four kinds of information received by muscle and tendon efferents: (1) muscle length, which is signaled by sensory endings on the intrafusal muscle fibers; (2) tension exerted by the muscle on the tendon, which is signaled by sensory endings (these sensory endings are within the Golgi tendon organ within the muscle-tendon junction (Figure 12.7); (3) deep pressure exerted upon muscles, which is signaled by Pacinian corpuscles contained within the membranous covering of the muscle or fascia; and (4) pain that accompanies prolonged exertion or muscle cramps; which is signaled by free nerve endings that follow the blood supply and are found throughout the muscle in its overlying fascia. During your yoga practice, you will experience the first three kinds of information received by your muscle and tendon efferents.

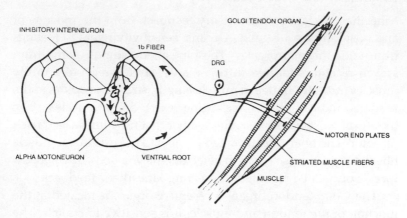

FIGURE 12.7 The Golgi tendon organ

The tissue that lines the joints contains free nerve endings and encapsulated receptors. The free nerve endings produce pain; the encapsulated receptors (such as Pacinian corpuscles) are sensitive to joint movement and position. Pacinian corpuscles and free nerve endings are also found in outer layers of various internal organs. They give rise to organic sensations. These sensations are much more subtle than the kinesthetic sensations. Nevertheless, you will from time to time feel the effects of your yoga practice on internal organ activities. An example of this would be increased gastrointestional activities following a shift toward parasympathetic nervous system dominance. This is sometimes the result of yogic meditative and relaxation practices.

Kinesthesia

In general, we should be aware that changes in the neuromuscular system automatically create change in our consciousness. Muscles do not act in isolation along a one-way track; rather, every muscular movement stimulates sensory cells within the muscles and tendons that "feed back" information to the brain's motor neurons, confirming their action. This loop system of the sensorimotor circuit guarantees that our brain is constantly receiving kinesthetic sensations of the ongoing state of the muscle system.

If the ongoing state of the muscles is tense, then the sensory cells will send a flood of feedback signals to bombard the brain. If the ongoing state of the muscles is relaxed, then the sensory cells will reduce their feedback signals down to a trickle. This leaves the brain free to notice and concentrate on other matters. Not only is one's awareness of the outer world less cloudy and distracted, so is one's awareness of one's inner somatic world. Proprioceptive awareness of oneself is an avenue of access to an immense realm of experience. Many of the descriptions of special states of mind attained in the advanced yogic practices are understandable only if one has sufficient internal proprioceptive awareness to understand these descriptions for what they are: special somatic states.

Although yoga was the ancient tradition to open the world of proprioceptive experience to exploration, this tradition has continued into the present time, taking on new forms: e.g., the Sensory Awareness teachings of Charlotte Selver, the delicate Eutony practices of Gerda Alexander and the Awareness Through Movement exercises of Moshe Feldenkrais.

Motor Cortex (Figure 12.8)

The area of the cortex most obviously involved in yoga's physical practices is the motor cortex (Figure 12.8). The motor cortex is the precentral gyrus — it is the fold of the cortex anterior to the central fissure. There is a motor "homunculus" located there (Figure 12.9). What is an homunculus? It is a mapping of the body proportionate to the amount of motor control to that area. The map can be explored during brain surgery; indeed, it frequently must be explored in order to be precise about surgical locations. You are mapped on your motor cortex upside down. There is a greater surface of the cortex devoted to areas of the body that require fine motor control; hands, fingers, etc. The motor cortex also shares neurons with the somatosensory cortex.

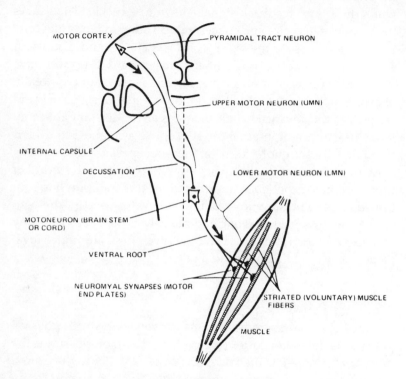

FIGURE 12.8 The motor cortex

The Somatosensory Cortex

Following yoga postures, you will feel sensations which result from somatosensory cortical activity. The somatosensory cortex is the postcentral gyrus. On the fold posterior to the central fissure, we have another upside-down map of the body (Figure 12.10). It has a greater territory devoted to areas of the body which have a

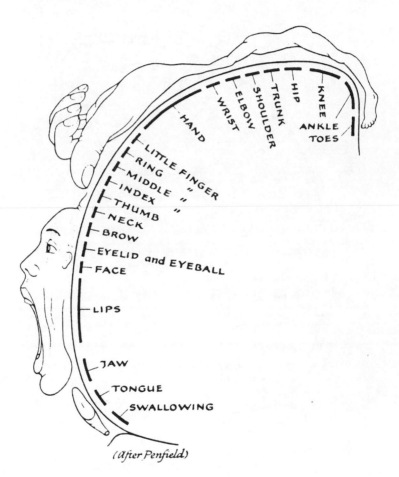

FIGURE 12.9 The motor homunculus

greater sensitivity. Lips and tongue, for example, have a dispro-
portionate area devoted to their sensory reception.

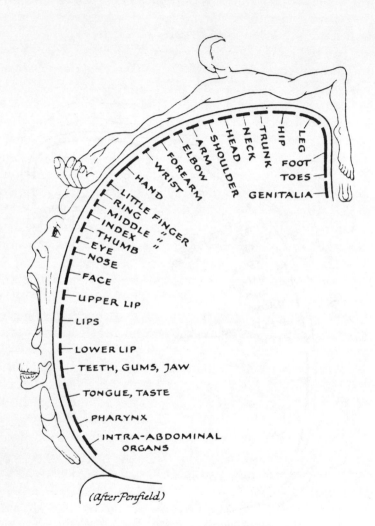

(after Penfield)

FIGURE 12.10 The sensory homunculus

As you are doing your asanas you are stimulating the sensori-motor cortex. As you move into the posture you have one kind of stimulation. As you maintain the posture you would be repeat-edly stimulating the same area of the sensorimotor cortex: you will stimulate the area that corresponds to the body's configuration. After you complete the posture you experience the sensations processed by the sensory cortex.

Here you have a loop which begins with visualizing the posture. The parietal-occipital-temporal (POT) area of the right hemisphere is probably activated by this. Then voluntary movement is initiated by areas which influence the motor cortex. From the pathways descending to the muscles comes the proper integrated information for contraction of the appropriate muscles. Finally, ascending pathways bring the information to the sensory cortex which again informs the motor cortex. Here we follow the same pattern as with concentration-meditation. If you focus attention on the sensory input modality, if you repeatedly suggest this event, then you move beyond a fragmented experience to one of integration and union. This experience is maintained for a finite period of time.

The reduction in the total amount of movement of the body suggests things to the reticular activating and thalamic activating systems. The slow, deliberate nature of the movements suggests things to the basal ganglia. All of these things help to set a special tone for the nervous system; they help shift toward parasympathetic nervous system dominance. They help maintain homeostasis. This uses the body's best handle, the neuromuscular system. The ultimate aim is toward a harmony among all the systems.

Psychophysiological research on hatha yoga has included electromyograph (EMG) studies and studies of flexibility measures. Recording the electrical activity of muscles is called electromyography (EMG). The electrical activity of muscles can be recorded from the surface of the skin or with needle electrodes. EMG measurements of yogic asanas are done by monitoring the activity, such as the degree of contraction or relaxation, of muscle groups.

Funderburk (1977) reports a study of a group of physical education teachers in India. They had practiced yoga asanas as part of their training; they were asked to do some of them while focusing on the infinite. Results showed that they were able to increase the degree of relaxation of the muscles involved. They were also able to extend the amount of time they were able to hold each posture comfortably and this increased the benefits of the posture.

K. S. Gopal and others (1975) compared two groups of subjects for six months. One group had trained in yoga previously, the other had no yoga training, but had done light exercises. As might be hypothesized, the EMG recordings were higher for the non-trained group. The corpse position was found to require the least muscular activity.

Flexibility

V. Hubert Dhanaraj randomly assigned 51 male college students to the 5 BX Program for Physical Fitness, a yoga group, or a control group (Dhanaraj, 1974). After six weeks of daily practice, the yoga group showed the greatest increase in flexibility, as measured by the Wells Sit-and-Reach Test.

Robson Moses (1972) measured changes in extension-flexion ranges of the left ankle, hip, hip and trunk, and neck. His subjects were 27 male physical education university students in the experimental and control groups. They were measured before and after 10 weeks of hatha yoga or physical education classes. Statistical analysis of the results showed a significant increase in flexibility for the hip, hip and trunk and neck for the yoga group. The ankle did not show the significant increases.

In somatic yoga, it is important to know as much as possible about how the asanas work physiologically. Not only is it important to do the postures, but also it is valuable to be aware of what is happening within the body. Mind is integrated with body. This will enable you to get maximum benefit from doing postures, increase mind/body integration, and transform the postures into meditative experiences.

13

The Senses and Concentration Training

*For me, my yoga is like my music and my dancing. It represents
a kind of freedom for me. I see yoga as a form of art as much as
a form of science. With yoga, as with dance, my body becomes alive.*

Yoga student

Concentration training is a way of stimulating your
senses. The cranial nerves are the primary sensory input channels
to your brain (Figure 13.1). Not only does yoga provide muscular
experiences, but also sensory stimulation for each of these channels. This way of looking at it enables us to understand the ratio-
nale for some of the practices. Let's look at the cranial nerves to see
how they are used by various yogic practices. The cranial nerves,
afferent pathways, are the sensory avenues bringing information
to the brain. How do they function? The following is a list of the
cranial nerves and yoga practices which stimulate them.

CN I–Olfactory (incense)

CN II–Optic (visual meditations)

CN III–Oculomotor (eye movement exercises; eye positions)

CN IV–Trochlear (eye movement; eye positions)

CN V–Trigeminal (the lion)

CN VI–Abducens (eye movements; eye positions)

CN VII–Facial (the lion)

CN VIII–Stato-acoustic (unusual balancing positions; auditory meditations, chanting)

CN IX–Glossopharyngeal (tastes; the lion pose)

CN X–Vagus (various postures)

CN XI–Spinal accessory (various postures)

CN XII–Hypoglossal (the lion)

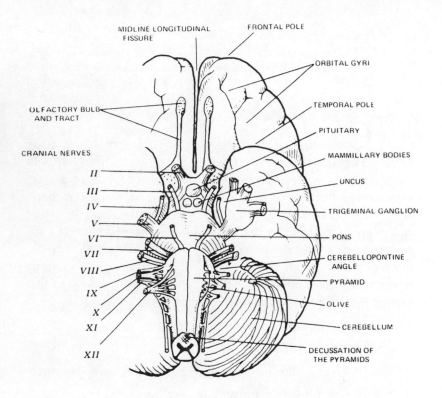

FIGURE 13.1 The cranial nerves.
(Modified from drawing by Lena Lyons.)

The vagus nerve, the longest cranial nerve, conveys fibers of the parasympathetic nervous system to organs of the thoracic and abdominal cavities. It also carries nonpainful sensory fibers back to the brain. The vagus nerve has been suggested as the possible site of kundalini pathway of yoga (see Ch. 14).

The Sensory Receptors

When energy from the environment impinges on a sensory receptor, that energy is transduced, changed into electrochemical impulses which travel along the sensory nerves. Sensory transduction is "the process by which sensory stimuli are transduced into slow, graded generator potentials or receptor potentials" (Carlson, 1977, p. 622). This means that energy in one form is translated into another form by the sensory receptor. Not only does each sense transduce energy, each sense accomplishes this in a different way. Then comes sensory coding. Sensory coding creates a representation of sensory events in the form of neural activity. As you concentrate on a meditation target, for example, you are stimulating one of your sensory receptors.

First let's look at receptor and generator potentials. A specialized neuron that serves as a receptor cell and produces a graded electrical potential is called a generator potential. The receptor potential is a slow, graded, electrical potential produced in response to a physical stimulus. Some receptor cells are neurons; some are not. Receptor potentials alter the firing rate of neurons upon which the receptors synapse.

A sensory modality refers to a particular form of sensory input. These include vision or audition or olfaction. That the somatosenses refer to bodily sensations seems clear. Sensitivity to touch, pain, and temperature are examples.

Sensory systems need to be used in order for their organic integrity to be maintained. Yoga provides a variety of stimulation for different parts of the sensory system.

Visual System (Figure 13.2)

When you are using a visual meditation target, you are stimulating the visual system. Let's look at how that occurs. The stimulus for vision is made up of light photons which impact on the retina. These are small packets of energy. The eyes are suspended in the orbits and are moved by six muscles that are attached to the sclera.

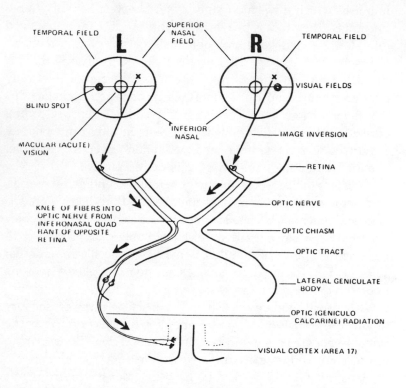

FIGURE 13.2 The visual system

The sclera is the outercoat of the eye. Folded back to attach to the eye, the conjunctiva are mucous membranes that line the eyelid. The cornea is a transparent, light-admitting layer of the pupil. The iris is one ring of muscles situated behind the cornea. The pupil — an expandable opening — is enlarged by the dilator muscle. The sphincter muscle, controlled by the parasympathetic nervous system, reduces the pupil when it contracts. The lens is behind the iris. The shape of the lens is controlled by the ciliary muscles. A kind of neural tissue, photoreceptive cells make up the retina located on the inner surface of the posterior of the eye. What is its function? Behind the pupil, it is the light receptive surface. The posterior chamber is the fluid-filled part of the eye.

The photoreceptors are the receptor cells of the retina. They transduce photoenergy into electrical potentials. The rods and cones are photoreceptors. The rods are "maximally sensitive to light of the same wave length" (Carlson, 1977, p. 620). They do not encode color vision. Just as the cones are maximally sensitive to one of three different wave lengths of light, so too they encode color vision. When you are using a particular meditation target, you are repeatedly stimulating an area of the rods and/or cones.

The fovea is the most sensitive portion of the retina: it is made up of a densely packed group of cones. This is where you generally sense the meditation target. The optic disk is formed by the point where fibers of the ganglion cells exit from the retina; the optic nerve also exits here. It is the "blind spot." The bipolar cell layer is made up of bipolar neurons that have only two processes: a dendritic process at one end and an axonal process at the other end.

Your use of the visual meditation target is, first of all, a biochemical event. Light reflected from your meditation target contacts your retina. The transduction of visual information occurs when photons (particles of energy making up light) impinge on the retinal cells. Paradoxically, light may be seen as electromagnetic radiation or as particles of energy. The photopigment is a special chemical including opsin, a protein. There is a series of chemical changes; retinal, a smaller molecule derived from Vitamin A, participates in the visual process. It is a molecule with a long chain and is capable of bending at a specific point. It consists of rod opsin plus retinal. All-transretinal is a straight-chained form of retinal; 11-cis-retinal is the bent form of all-transretinal. Malleable, 11-cis-retinal is the only naturally occurring form of retinal capable of attaching to rod opsin to form rhodopsin. Thus, you can see the complex biochemical series which you begin when you observe the light of your meditation target.

Within the visual system we have a spatial representation of the world due to the mosaic representation of the retina. Passed from the retina to the occipital lobe is a spatial representation with a point-by-point representation. The representation on the cortex of the retinal mosaic has been called retinotopic. The fovea, central region of the retina, is 25% of the visual cortex. Transduced, information enters the visual system and bifurcates (forks into two branches) at the optic chiasm (Figure 13.2). The retinotectal tract is the pathway from the retina to the superior colliculi. The superior colliculi is located in the tectal region of the brainstem or the midbrain, if you remember. So you can see that part of the information from your meditation target goes to the primitive visual area of the brainstem.

The secondary visual cortex surrounds the primary cortex; it is responsible for the first level of making the sensation meaningful to you.

Auditory System

The stimulus for hearing is 20–15,000 Hz (cycles per second). When you use an auditory meditation target, you are selecting a sound that is within that frequency range.

Figure 13.3 shows the anatomy of the ear. The external ear is called the pinna. From the outside we can see the external auditory canal. The tympanic membrane is the ear drum. Called the tensor tympani, the muscle, attached to the malleus, contracts tensing the tympanic membrane. Within are the ossicles, the bones of the middle ear. They include the malleus, the incus, and the stirrups. The base plate of the stapes presses against a membrane across the oval window. The base plate transmits sound vibrations into the fluid within the cochlea, a snail-shaped structure. The oval window is an opening in the bone surrounding the cochlea.

The sound from your meditation target enters the chochlea in the inner ear. The cochlea contains the auditory transducing mechanisms which transduce the sound vibrations from your meditation target into electrochemical impulses. The cochlea has

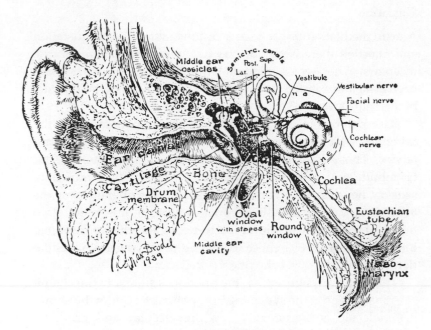

FIGURE 13.3 The anatomy of the ear. (After Brodel, 1939)
(Garoutte, 1987, p. 118)

two-and-three-quarter turns. It also contains hair cells, which have a key function: they are the receptive cells of the auditory or vestibular apparatus.

The activity begun by the vibrations of your meditation target is translated into electrochemical impulses which travel along the auditory nerve.

The auditory nerve has two branches: the cochlear nerve and the vestibular nerve. The nerve impulses which relate to hearing travel along the cochlear nerve to areas of the brain responsible for processing auditory information. The vestibular nerve transmits impulses to the vestibular system, which helps us process information about our body's position in space. Yoga postures give ample stimulation to the vestibular nerve.

Gustation

A taste meditation target uses a unique system. With gustation and olfaction there is no obvious transmission of energy to the receptors. When we examine the stimuli in a simple way, as has been done historically, we can see the following qualities of taste: bitter, salty, sweet, sour.

The point of contact for a taste meditation focus is the tastebuds which are found in the tongue, palate, pharynx, and larynx. These taste receptors—there are approximately 10,000 taste buds—are specialized cells that synapse with dendrites of sensory neurons. The papillae are small protruberances of the tongue; they have moat-like trenches surrounding them. Two hundred taste buds surround the trenches and their pores open into the trench. The chemical combination of your taste meditation target washes over the open pores.

Transduction of gustatory information is similar to the chemical transmission at the synapses. Some characteristic of the stimulus molecule is "recognized" by the receptor and produces changes in membrane permeability and subsequent receptor potentials. Electrochemical impulses are transmitted then through the nervous system.

The routes of the gustatory fibers to the brain are originated by cell bodies located in CN VII Facial, IX Glossopharyngeal, X Vagus (pharynx and throat) nerves.

Olfaction

Information from your olfactory meditation target uses a chemical stimulus. The stimulus for the olfactory system consists of the molecules of substances that are volatile (they evaporate at a reasonable temperature). They dissolve in the mucous that coats the olfactory epithelium.

The molecules from your meditation target (incense, for example) are actually inhaled. They are then dissolved at the olfactory epithelium level. The anatomy of the olfactory apparatus begins with the olfactory receptors that reside in two patches of olfactory epithelium. These are located in the mucous membrane at the top of your nasal cavity. The turbinate bones—bony ridges—are bones that help sweep the air up to reach the sensory receptors. From the end of the olfactory nerve are the protrusions which form the olfactory bulbs. They receive input from the olfactory receptors. The cribriform plate is the bony plate below the olfactory bulb. The axons pass through the cribriform plate. Also, the trigeminal fibers terminate here to mediate pain arising from noxious chemical stimulation.

The anatomy of the olfactory receptors indicates that the receptors are cell bodies of neurons: their axons pass through the cribriform plate. Cilia on the receptors project from the surface of the mucosa.

The olfactory information of your meditation target is transduced in a mysterious way. How the generator potential is produced by the odor molecules of your meditation target stimulating the cilia at the receptor sites is not known. Mitral cells in the olfactory bulbs are synapsed on by axons of the olfactory receptors. The olfactory glomeruli are complex axonic and dendritic aborizations: some axons synapse in the brain, others cross the brain and enter the other olfactory nerve and synapse in the contralateral olfactory bulb. The electrochemical impulses produced travel to the rhinencephalon, the "smell brain," where the information is processed.

The human nose can differentiate about seven primary odors. The seven primary odors detectable include: camphoracious, ethereal, floral, musky, pepperminty, pungent, and putrid (Carlson, 1977, p. 246). Your olfactory meditation target will be composed of one or more of these odors.

As you do your concentration practice, you repeatedly stimulate sensory receptors. The sensory receptors stimulated—visual, auditory, olfactory—depend on the meditation target you have selected. The sensory receptor then transduces (translates) the information from its original form of energy into electrochemical impulses. These impulses travel along the nerve pathways; the pathways are specific to that sensory mode. Specific areas of the cortex are repeatedly stimulated by the electrochemical impulses. The reticular activating system is also stimulated. This process is continued for as long as you attend to that target — as long as you stimulate that sensory system. The longer you maintain your concentration, the more likely you are to experience a physiological shift into the next state.

The next state includes a shift toward parasympathetic nervous system dominance. The PNS is part of the autonomic nervous system.

Autonomic Nervous System (Figure 13.4)

The autonomic nervous system — portions of the peripheral nervous system that regulate the vegetative functions — has two branches (Figure 13.4). The two branches are the sympathetic and parasympathetic nervous systems. The sympathetic (fight or flight) system, mediates functions that accompany arousal. It is basically catabolic — concerned with the breakdown of stored energy. The parasympathetic is anabolic and mediates functions that occur during the relaxed state.

The sympathetic nervous system changes include an increase in blood pressure, heart rate, respiration rate, brainwave frequencies, etc. The sympathetic nervous system, a more unitary system than the parasympathetic nervous system, is composed of a ganglionic chain that parallels the spinal cord. The neurons synapse here and extend to the organ or gland they innervate.

The parasympathetic nervous system is sometimes considered the reciprocal of the sympathetic nervous system; it counteracts the effects of the sympathetic nervous system. Its neurons leave the central nervous system at the brainstem and caudal portion of the spinal cord. It extends to the same organs and glands as the sympathetic nervous system except for the smooth muscles of the peripheral blood vessels, the sweat glands of the hands and feet and the piloerector muscles in the skin. It is the system concerned with maintenance and repair and it is particularly affected by your yoga practice.

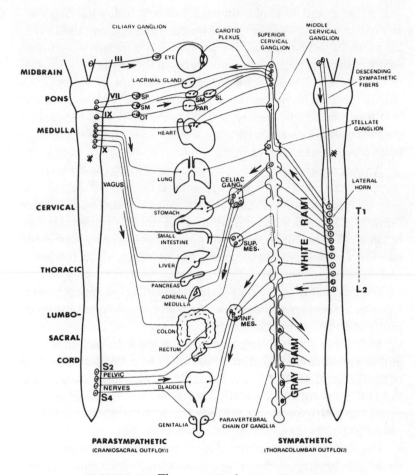

FIGURE 13.4 The autonomic nervous system

To a large extent the gradually ascending stages of yoga represent a gradual cultivation of dominance in the parasympathetic system. The distracting and energy-wasting anxieties of the sympathetic mode are suppressed, leaving consciousness free and clear of the "monkey of the mind" alarms caused by the fight-or-flight drives.

This conquest of the sympathetic nervous functions is obvious in the hatha yoga level of training. Obtaining full, voluntary control of the neuromuscular system means overcoming the keyed-up tonus of tight muscles that automatically occurs with dominance of the sympathetic system. Beneath the impressive suppleness and body control achieved by the hatha practitioner is the simple fact that he or she has learned to contract muscles at will and totally relax them at will. This is the ability to maintain a parasympathetic state which evokes slower, more rhythmical brain waves and a calmer mind.

Another example of this gain in parasympathetic dominance occurs in pranayama, when the breathing is disciplined. Pranayama exercises create a growing voluntary control of the mechanics of breathing. Inasmuch as air is, along with nutrition, the main sustenance of life and of all metabolic process, we can be sure that full control of breathing has the profoundest effects upon the entire central nervous system.

To mention but one aspect of this: deep, diaphragmatic breathing overcomes sympathetic dominance of heart function, dropping the rate of heart beat and blood pressure and creating a soft, up and down rhythm that accelerates a little during inhalation and slows during exhalation. This calm and healthy heartbeat occurs because diaphragmatic breathing brings more oxygen into the blood stream. Additionally, the up and down heart rhythm sends constantly varying pressures through the entire cardiovascular system, keeping it supple.

The sheer ability to breath deeply into the diaphragm evokes all of the healthful effects of maintenance and repair of the parasympathetic nervous system. That in itself is enough. But when we include the fact that we experience calmness and greater ease, we see how this healthy somatic state fits into the yogic desire for a higher consciousness.

In somatic yoga, it is important to remember the anatomy and physiology involved in the practices. It would be valuable for you to learn the material in this chapter, if you do not already know it, so that you could keep it in mind as you do your yoga practice.

PART FIVE

The Spiritual Side of Somatic Yoga

14

Somatic Yoga, Altered States of Consciousness, and the Kundalini Experience

When these three—concentration, meditation and absorption—are brought to bear upon one subject, they are called samyama.

Through mastery of samyama comes the light of knowledge.

Patanjali

My yoga has begun to take a fairly regular and graceful state. I find myself practicing joyfully because I want to. Yoga is enhancing to my daily life activities and I feel its effects on my consciousness and vibration. I feel centered under circumstances where before I practiced yoga I felt uncentered.

I feel greater endurance and especially greater body awareness and also a greater sensitivity to others.

Yoga student

When the environmental stimulation or internal stimulation change in intensity, increasing or decreasing, our nervous systems respond. We enter an altered nervous system state which has been called an altered state of consciousness (ASC) (Tart, 1975). Arnold M. Ludwig (1975, p. 12) defines altered states of consciousness (ASC) as "any mental state(s), induced by various physiological, psychological, or pharmacological maneuvers or agents, which can be recognized subjectively by the individual himself (or by an objective observer of the individual) as representing a sufficient deviation in subjective experience or psychological functioning from certain general norms for that individual during alert, waking consciousness." This change may be characterized by a greater awareness of internal sensations or mental processes, changes in quality of thought, and difficulty in reality testing.

An ASC may be produced by altering the normal flow of movements, sensory input, emotional expression, or cognitive processes. If you alter the adaptation level of stimulation of the person either above or below his adapted level, there will be a reaction.

Ludwig lists categories of variables that induce an ASC. These include: "A. Reduction of exteroceptive stimulation and/or motor activity; B. Increase of exteroceptive stimulation and/or motor activity and/or emotion; C. Increased alertness or mental involvement; and D. Decreased alertness or relaxation of critical faculties" (1975, p. 12).

Yoga practice utilizes the first category, "reduction of exteroceptive stimulation and/or motor activity," through reducing sensory input. Another characteristic of this category is the repetition of stimuli—yoga uses various means such as concentration training to provide this. Another is "a drastic reduction of motor activity." The example of this is sitting in meditation or holding a posture for an extended period of time.

The second category—"increase of exteroceptive stimulation and/or motor activity and/or emotion"—may be seen in the use of prolonged chanting and other dance-like movements sometimes done to music in a yogic setting. The increased alertness—mental involvement—may come after prolonged meditation and intense chanting. From passive meditation, when the samadhi experience occurs, may come decreased alertness.

The presence of somatopsychic factors may contribute to the ASC produced by yoga practice. When there are differences in oxygen present, when there are changes in the body's biochemistry, and perhaps even the production of endorphins (the brain's endogeneous morphine-like chemicals), there is a change in neurological functions.

The general characteristics of ASCs that Ludwig (1975, pp. 15–17) presents include: alterations in thinking; disturbed time sense;

loss of control; change in emotional expression; body image change; perceptual distortions; change in meaning or significance; sense of the ineffable; feelings of rejuvenation; and hypersuggestibility. Let's look at how these characteristics of the ASC relate to yoga experiences.

Alterations in Thinking

Examples of this include changes in your concentration, memory, and judgment. You may become less clear about cause and effect relationships; you may find paradoxical concepts easier to entertain.

Sense of Time

Your sense of time may become changed. Distorted, time may seem to go faster or slower. You may experience the "now" as being timeless. These distortions of time are usually temporary experiences.

Loss of Control

Loss of control in an ASC may be behavioral, emotional, or cognitive. It may have the opposite effect. Sometimes the person may experience difficulty in losing himself in the experience of deep meditation. How does this happen? There may be a lot of "ego chatter." Ego chatter includes a number of irrelevant thoughts which come incessantly into your mind while you are trying to clear your mind.

Emotional Expression

With your yoga practice you will experience a change in your emotional expression. You may feel intense happiness, intense love for all of humankind and nature – perhaps emotions like intense, joyous sadness. You may sometimes feel somewhat detached from human emotions; human events may take on a transcendent quality. You may also feel touched by cosmic humor.

Body Image

Ludwig lists a feeling of a change in body image. With yoga practice you may feel that your body is less burdensome to you than usual; it may feel lighter. You may feel a blurring of your physical boundaries so that you *do* feel one with the universe. You may feel various unusual body sensations such as a tingling or numbness.

Perceptions

Ludwig lists a category of perceptual distortions. Perceptual distortions are sensory illusions. You may experience sensory illusions, such as sound or lights, for which there are no external sources; you might also experience synesthesia. Synesthesia, a sensory mix, is the tendency to experience sensory input through another sense. Not only might you see a visual image, but also hear the image or vice versa.

Meaning

With yoga practice you may experience what Ludwig classifies as an intensification of meaning or the significance of experiences. You will find that ordinary experiences will become meaningful; you may find life becoming deeply meaningful in a cosmic sense.

The Ineffable

The classification of the sense of the ineffable refers to experiences that are beyond the capability of words to convey. Certainly yoga, a largely nonverbal experience, includes much that is beyond words. As you experience what seems like indentification with the Infinite, this experience is beyond words.

Rejuvenation

The yogic experience may lead you to a feeling of rejuvenation. A feeling of new excitement about the business of living and about yourself and others.

Hypersuggestibility

The state of hypersuggestibility which is a part of an ASC is also characteristic of the yogic experience. This kind of response among meditators to one another and to a leader or guru is part of the heightened awareness stage. Because of the hypersuggestibility, it is useful to give yourself what Mishra calls post-meditative suggestions, suggestions of attitudes or behaviors that are part of your next development. It is also important to use your good common sense in following suggestions given to you by others.

The positive use of the ASC listed by Ludwig (1975) include: (1) healing; (2) avenues of new knowledge or experience; and (3) social function. If we look at these uses, in the light of yoga, we see that through the centuries it has been considered a healing agent. From the insights that come to the person during and after meditation, we see the avenue of new knowledge. What is also found is the expanded knowledge available to you when you practice samyama on sources of knowledge that you value—persons, objects, and situations. The social function of yoga is that it has provided, in India, a socially approved possiblity for experiencing an ASC. In the West, it has become, for many people, an avenue for altering consciousness safely. It provides an expanded relationship to others and facilitates social interchange.

Environmental and internal stimulation levels are constantly changing in intensity. These changes sometimes reflect natural fluctuations such as circadian rhythms. "Circadian" comes from the Latin "circa." "Circa" means "approximate" or "about" and "dia" refers to day. These are biological changes that biological organisms experience during a 24-hour period. Some of the changes are induced changes, such as those produced by your actions or by others around you. As that stimulation changes, your nervous system activity changes in response to the stimuli. With your changes in nervous system activity come changes in levels of consciousness. One can at that point speak of an altered state of consciousness.

When you are in an altered state of consciousness you know it because of changes in your perceptions, sense of time, physiological sensations, and emotions different from what you might expect under other circumstances. It is the perception of the experience by you that heralds the altered state of consciousness.

There are a variety of means for altering one's consciousness. Some of these are natural, such as "highway hypnosis," sleep, and dreams; some are induced by actions that we deliberately take, such as drinking alcohol, fasting, etc.

Yoga is one excellent way to alter consciousness. It does it by altering the psychophysiological state and, therefore, the perceptual experience of the individual. At one time the change in consciousness afforded by yoga was considered permanent, but that is not true. As long as you do your yoga practice consistently, you will experience the change. If you cease to do your practice, your body will gradually recover its original state of stiffness and tension and you will cease to experience the world in the yogic way. When you resume your practice, in a relatively short time you will recover the state that you had achieved earlier.

From the prolonged practice of yoga, the body seems to go through an alchemical process that transmutes it into a system that can more easily conduct energy or what feels like "energy." At that time some individuals experience an increase in available energy. This activation of stored energy has been considered, in India, the energy of the kundalini.

The kundalini (coiled sepent power) is said to lie dormant at the base of the spine. As it is awakened, it seems to climb up the region of the spinal column or the sushumna through the chakras (energy vortices corresponding to the nerve plexuses of Western physiology) to the area of the third eye (center of the forehead between the eyebrows) or the location of Shakti. There a marriage of Shakti and Shiva is said to take place. That is the completion of the awakening process. Some yogas call for stimulating the kundalini more or less directly to hasten the awakening process. Other yogas, raja being one of them, call for it to happen naturally as an indirect result of the yogi's practice.

When the kundalini moves up the sushumna it is said that the chakras (energy vortices) open up. As they open, there is the sense that the capacities associated with those levels become more accessible.

The Chakras

Western writers correlate the chakras with nerve plexuses, ganglia, and glands. Eastern thinkers think of them as potential energy sources: transpersonal Being-energy is necessary to actualize their spiritual potential (Chaudhuri, 1975). The chakras do relate to the physiological systems, however.

Opening the root center (the first chakra, located at the base of the spine) means the "shifting of consciousness from the egocentric to the cosmo-centric or Being-centric focus" (Chaudhuri, 1975). The root center relates to the material world. Some have related it to the sacral plexus in the region of the anus; others, to the sacrococcygeal plexus mid-way between the genitals and anus.

The instinctual center (second chakra) relates to the prostatic or epigastric plexus. Not only is it related to the nerve plexus, but also it is related to the gonads. When the kundalini reaches this center, there is an upsurge of sexual energy. Here one experiences Being as vital energy, one experiences the transcendent state.

The third chakra "is the center of higher ambition and the will to power." Some feel the naval center relates to the solar plexus; others, to the lumbar plexus. The naval center, the center of the body, relates to the adrenal gland. This is also a dangerous level as one feels the strength of the will to power and may identify with it.

The fourth chakra "is the center of the soul or psychic being." It is the seat of unselfish love—it is the seat of the sense of higher values. Here one experiences spiritual love. This is a love that is unconditional love. It may be directed toward humans or the Supreme. It is a spontaneous and intrinsically joyful state; one also hears the nad sound in this state. This sound—it is the music of the spheres—was said to have been present at the beginning of creation. It is the original sound. It has been equated with the higher Self: the part of you that observes your behavior. It relates to the cardiac plexus and the thymus gland.

The fifth chakra "is the center of pure and distinctive awareness of things as they are in their uniqueness or suchness." It is the throat chakra. It relates to the pharyngeal or laryngeal plexus and thyroid gland. It facilitates concentration, intense self-projection, intuition.

The sixth chakra is the wisdom center or divine command center or the third eye of philosophic knowledge. It relates to the cavernous plexus. A rudimentary light sensing organ, this is related to the pineal gland. Some associate it with the pituitary gland or the cerebellum. The center of spiritual enlightment, it has its own authority. It has the power of self-fulfillment. What happens when you "open the third eye?" In opening it you gain self-mastery. You, transformed, experience the unconditional imperative of your higher Self. It is the imperative of your own destiny, the freely chosen mission of your life.

The seventh chakra, the highest center, the crown center, has been called the thousand-petaled lotus. "It is the center of genuine transcendental consciousness. It relates to the top of the skull or upper brain." It also relates to the pituitary gland. "On attainment of this level of consciousness a person gains enormous power for healing people and making them whole by transmitting the power of illumined and integrated consciousness. It is the experience of oneness with the non-temporal Being" (Chaudhuri, 1975).

Opening the Third Eye

The third eye is said to be located in the center of the forehead. It is triangular in shape; it represents eternal knowledge. It is considered not only a physiological location, but also a psychic chakra by yogis. Ordinarily it is said to be functioning only partially—its function awaits awakening. As we learn more it becomes more fully functioning. Yoga—a practice designed to awaken it—allows it to begin to function perfectly. Awakening this chakra is called opening the third eye: it is not an anatomical eye. At a different evolutionary level, some other animals do have a third eye which is in conjunction with the pineal gland. Just as for those animals there is a light sensitive area at the top of the head, so too this area gives information to the pineal body. In humans, the third eye is called an eye by yogis—through its perceptions we see our own true nature and that of the world around us. To open the third eye you must know anatomy, physiology and yoga psychology.

The steps toward opening the third eye include: 1) place your body in a comfortable position; 2) clear your mind; 3) recognize the ocean of energy in which your body is resting; 4) practice pratyahara (withdraw energy from your body and place it on the area of the third eye. Practice samyama on that place. Listen to the nad sound); 5) remain in this state until you forget your body. You will begin to identify with supreme consciousness. At this point you will experience the highest intuition and penetrating will power. Practice this repeatedly going as far as you can with each experience.

Some of the experiences reported by persons in the kundalini awakening state are suggestive of psi. The relationship of somatic yoga to psychic experiences is the subject of our next chapter.

15

Somatic Yoga and Psi

The psychic powers may be obtained either by birth, or by means of drugs, or by the power of words, or by the practice of austerities, or by concentration.

Patanjali

My yoga is loose and seemingly discontinuous. I go through experience sometimes asleep, sometimes awake, dreaming and perceiving "normally," and my yoga is the thread being pulled through it all attaching the subconscious to the conscious. It seems slow but is growing exponentially in that I'm able to grasp – more and more threads in the twilight space between and they continue to intertwine and strengthen themselves. It is loose, long and consumes me.

Yoga student

Altered states of consciousness have been found to be psi-conducive states of consciousness. What this means is that during an ASC you are more likely to have an experience suggestive of psi than during ordinary states of consciousness. The practice of somatic yoga encourages the experience of altered states of consciousness. As discussed in earlier chapters, the practices of yoga alter your psychophysiological state. Therefore, the nervous system of the individual is affected. With meditation there is frequently a shift in brain waves to alpha (8–12 Hz) and sometimes to theta (4–7 Hz). There has been some evidence that there is a correlation between alpha and theta and psi.

Psi is a term that has been used to refer to psychic ability in general. There are four categories of psi: telepathy, clairvoyance, precognition, and psychokinesis. A mysterious phenomenon, telepathy refers to the transmission of information without known channels of information transfer. Clairvoyance refers to knowing about situations or objects without the aid of human intermediaries, i.e., there is no one living who knows the information, therefore, no one can give the information telepathically. To qualify as genuine, precognition—knowing about future events before they happen—needs proof that the knowledge was not acquired by ordinary means. Psychokinesis is a different sort of ability or tendency. It refers to impacting on material objects and events without touching them.

There are a couple of ways to look at the theories which attempt to explain the reality of psi. Lawrence LeShan spelled them out neatly in his *Toward a General Theory of the Paranormal* (1969) and *The Medium, the Mystic, and the Physicists* (1973). He used two approaches to classify them. One approach had to do with energy or information transmission through space; the other had to do with a merging of fields of consciousness. In the latter, there was an instantaneous transmission of information between the merged fields because they were unified. The latter is suggestive of the unification experience of samadhi.

There is another aspect of yoga practice which is significant. The fact that yoga is non-verbal and deals particularly with the body indicates a shift to right hemisphere dominance. From right hemisphere research comes the possibility that the right hemisphere is associated with the unconscious and intuitive perceptions. The unconscious has been called the royal road of psi.

In yoga it has been considered important not to focus on paranormal abilities. They are to be used as part of one's development. Since the stage of psi phenomena seems to be just below the stage of enlightenment, it is considered a trap in which one might get stuck. Fascinated with the paranormal phenomena, one might not be able to get beyond them to a higher goal.

There have been many claims in India of persons with paranormal abilities. There have been many claims that yoga can be used to develop those abilities, perceptions, tendencies. For the ordinary person a little psychic development might be helpful, but not too much. How it can be helpful is seen in examples such as increases in empathic ability, some sense of the precognitive aspect of dreams, some telepathic sense of the thoughts of others for increased understanding (see Table 1).

The yoga experience creates a psi-conductive state. Although psychic experiences are not automatic, they are more likely to occur. We can say that during a period of sustained yoga practice you might experience more psychic experiences; more experiences will be suggestive of psi than during a period of abstinence from yoga practice. What you can assume is that they are a by-product of your experience. Yoga seems to creat a psychophysiological state in which psi is more possible than it is in our ordinary psychophysiological state.

With yoga practice, psi experiences are likely to come in precognitive or telepathic forms. Being vividly aware, you are more likely to experience telepathic understandings from other people. You will frequently experience flashes of insight about your own activities, self, future; you may experience meditative understandings that are beyond the range of information that is ordinarily available to you.

Paranormal abilities that have been traditionally reported by yogis include entering into other bodies, telepathy, doing things according to one's own will, clairvoyance, clairaudience, omniscience, effulgence, vanishing from sight at will, and still others. The miraculous ability to enter into the bodies of others is said to be part of why the early Indians had such an advanced understanding of the human body. Clairvoyance (clear seeing) is the capacity to know about distant objects or situations without a human intermediary. Clairaudience refers to hearing at a distance. Omniscience, knowledge that has no boundary, stands for all knowing. Effulgence is the tendency to glow. This occurs in certain psychophysiological states reported by yogis, particularly those of ecstacy. The capacity to vanish from sight at will is the capacity to handle one's body and matter in a way that changes the viewer's perceptions. And there are others.

You can use psi as a natural part of your yogic development. By letting yoga help you ralate to your world from a state of union, you do not experience the usual sense of separateness. The

Table 1. *Powers Produced by Full Meditation*

1. Knowledge of the past and future
2. Understanding of sounds made by all creatures
3. Knowledge of past lives
4. Knowing what others are thinking
5. Prior knowledge of one's death
6. Attainment of various kinds of strength
7. Perception of the small, the concealed, and the distant
8. Knowledge of other inhabited regions
9. Knowledge about the stars and their motions
10. Knowledge of the interior of the body
11. Control of hunger and thirst
12. Steadiness
13. Seeing the adepts in one's own interior light
14. Entering the bodies of others
15. Lightness and levitation
16. Brightness
17. Control of material elements
18. Control of the senses
19. Perfection of the body
20. Quickness of the body, and the well-known set of eight powers
    (1.) Minuteness: to be as small as an atom at will
    (2.) Expansion: to increase in size at will
    (3.) Lightness: neutralization of gravity at will
    (4.) Reaching: to obtain anything or to reach any place at will
    (5.) Acquirement: to have the fulfillment of any wish at will
    (6.) Lordship: control of the energies of nature at will
    (7.) Self-control: self-command and freedom from being influenced at will
    (8.) Desire-control: the stopping of all desires at will

From *Yoga* by Ernest Wood, Penguin Books Ltd., 1962, pp. 78–79.

insights can be used as guidance: the information is then reviewed with your critical mind to validate its appropriateness. Psi can be used as a cue to let you know when you are on the path that is right for you.

In the *Yoga Sutras* by Patanjali, the main way of developing paranormal abilities is through the process of samyama. The process of samyama has three parts: (1) fixation of attention on the object or person of interest (concentration); (2) meditation or entering into a loop with the meditation target; and (3) union with the object of meditation for a period of time. As we enter union with the meditation target, not only do we blend with it, but we can also, therefore, share knowledge with it. When we leave the state of union, we take with us the memory of having been one. "One knows the inmost cause of things and one reaches the great light of wisdom."

Extrasensory perception is an outgrowth of concentration practice. As you practice yoga you will be able to perceive sensory input above and below the usual thresholds. Mishra (1959) says that one aim of yoga is to examine all sensory input: you must increase the impact of all sensations up to the level of perception. It is important to know the anatomy and physiology of the senses. Through concentration practices you can expand your range of perception. If you expand your perceptual range, you will be more able to experience an expanded reality.

Extrasensory perception is not a function of the senses, it is a function of consciousness. From the extrasensory experiences of yoga come contributions to the development of the person.

Mishra (1959) says that in order to develop extrasensory perception it is valuable to meditate on nadam, the subtle vibratory sound. Along with this one would practice tratakam (concentration training) on the appropriate target. Mishra felt that the paranormal powers were acquired in the following ways: (1) by birth; (2) by chemical means; (3) by mantra and study; (4) by self-discipline and removal of ego self; and (5) by samadhi and concentration. These ways he explained as follows. Some individuals, and families, seem to be genetically predisposed to psychic sensitivities: that is, certain people, environment permitting, seem to be more prone from birth to such experiences. "Chemical means" refers to certain drugs–marijuana and LSD–that have been reported to yield perceptions suggestive of paranormal experiences. By "mantra and study," Mishra, a great believer in the repetition of mantras, refers to the effect of repetition on the nervous system. The effect of increased knowledge through the study of classic yogic literature on openess to experience might also be noticed. "Self-discipline and removal of ego self" would enable you to control the self, to remove the ego boundaries which separate you from direct knowing. "Samadhi and concentration" refer to the unification experience and the concentration that leads to it. The first four approaches are considered secondary and temporary; the fifth, primary and permanent.

We can look at the claims of spontaneous psi in yoga from the perspective of modern parapsychology and see what our understanding might be. Although you may experience spontaneous events suggestive of psi, parapsychologists are trying to do controlled studies which take into consideration the many ways that information can leak through to us through non-psychic means.

In 1934 J. B. Rhine published a monograph entitled *Extra Sensory Perception*. This was an overview of his experiments at Duke University which began in 1927 and were far more systematic than earlier parapsychological studies. As with any research tradition, his studies became more rigorous as they evolved. Criticisms from other researchers suggested possibilities for tightening controls.

Parapsychology is a branch of science that is concerned with ESP and PK. ESP is extrasensory perception, perception beyond our ordinary senses. PK (psychokinesis) is a behavioral or personal exchange with the environment: it does not use our sensorimotor system in order to create its effects.

Extrasensory perception is usually considered to entail three different abilities. These abilities are: telepathy (which is communication from mind to mind outside the regular sensory channels); clairvoyance (the perception of situations from a distance, but not by way of a mind that may be perceiving the situation);

and precognition (foreknowledge of some future event). There is some dispute among researchers over whether these are separate processes or whether they may be explained one by the other. Precognition, although quite unusual from our consensually validated conception of time, is easier to research because the target has not yet been selected. It is, therefore, freer from obvious information leakage.

In parapsychological research we need to rule out chance factors as an explanation for events. Carl Jung presented the concept of synchronicity (1952), namely, an acausal meaningful coincidence that has an acausal connecting principle. If a coincidence is to qualify as synchronistic, there needs to be a coming together of two events plus an observer. The observer helps experience the meaningfulness of the connection.

In paranormal research there is an attempt to assure that the results are statistically significant, that they could not have happened by chance. In order to insure that the results could not have happened by chance, parapsychologists use a significance level which is even more rigorous that that used in other areas of psychological research: the .001 significance level. This means that the results would only have happened by chance one in 1,000 times.

ESP has been defined as "information obtained by a person about an event without the use of known means of information." In order to "prove" ESP in a laboratory study, all possible information leaks must be controlled. In spontaneous psi events such as in yoga experiences, it is sometimes difficult to determine whether there is any possible information available through known means.

In parapsychological research the term, "psi-conducive states of consciousness," has been used to refer to a special state of consciousness, usually an altered state, in which psychic experiences are more likely to occur.

In parapsychology, the term, field consciousness (FC), has been used to describe the person experiencing an enlargement of self-boundaries: with an expanded sense of self the environment may seem to merge with his sense of self. This is suggestive of the samadhi experience.

Psi-hitting is a situation in which, during paranormal research, you are able to guess correctly the intended target. From psi-missing we can sometimes see psi ability unconsciously avoiding the target. What it shows is the cleverness of sensing what the target is and, unconsciously, deliberately avoiding it. Both psi-hitting and psi-missing reveal the presence of psi.

The sheep-goat effect is a term used to describe the observation that a belief in psi affects scoring levels (Schmeidler, 1974). Believers tend to have scores greater than those they would achieve through chance; those who do not believe in psi tend to score below chance. It seems as if the non-believer makes very sure, on an unconscious level, that he will not choose the correct answer.

Psi-mediated instrumental response (PMIR) is a term, developed by Rex Stanford (1972), that refers to responses of the organism (human or other) that help fulfill its needs. It requires a combination of psi factors such as ESP and/or PK; it requires a need on the part of the organism. The organism does not need to be intending or aware of the event occurring. PMIR is a possible explanation of the experience of a series of fortunate or unfortunate events, a run of good or bad luck. Sometimes when you notice a trend in events, a series of qualitatively similar situations, PMIR may be operating. If the events do not seem to further your development, through meditation and work on yourself, you can change the trend.

Some people who have practiced yoga have experienced out-of-the-body experiences. This is an experience in which you feel as though your "self" is located outside your physical body. Robert Monroe (1971) has written convincingly of his personal experiences with out-of-the-body travel. Complex experiences such as this are very challenging to parapsychological researchers.

Yoga practices and meditation have been considered psi-conducive. As you do your practice you may notice that synchronistic events happen more frequently. When you are not consistent in your yoga practice, they decrease. You may notice that you are more empathic about the emotions of others and that you are more aware of the thoughts of others. Sensing what is going to happen, you may even have more expanded knowledge of events. Your dreams may be seemingly more telepathic or precognitive.

One of the effects of yoga is the stimulation of primitive areas of the brain. MacLean (1973) says that we have three evolutionary levels present within our brains: (1) reptilian; (2) mammalian; (3) human. This has been called the triune brain. All levels are still functioning in balance with the later levels of development. The newer areas inhibit the older levels to a degree. It is probably the primitive areas of the brain that are implicated in psychic perception. Psychic perception seems more prevalent in children and animals. As our cortex becomes more developed with age— myelinization of neurons and connections of synapses in neural circuits—we no longer process that kind of information as reality. No more imaginary playmates.

Yoga uses a number of means to help us return to the more primitive levels of the brain. It is not that we wish to de-evolve; we merely wish to have access to all of our capacities and capabilities. Meditation, where cortical activity is decreased; incense, causing olfactory bulb stimulation and input to the rhinencephalon; postures representing animals; eye position gazes and input to the brain stem; breath regulation which drives the medulla—all are practices which seem to contribute to stimulating primitive areas of the brain.

Used properly, the psychic byproducts of yoga practice will aid your development and liberation. With a combination of pratyahara and samyama, physical culture is increased. With this combination the senses are heightened. Clairaudience and clairvoyance may indeed be possible.

If, as a byproduct of your yogic practice, you begin to experience what has been called paranormal experiences, do not be afraid of them. What you must do is grow used to them so that the expanded world-view becomes the comfortable one. For example, if you dream about the death of a loved one, this is cause for anguish. But if you see life and death as part of the balance of the universe, then the foreknowledge of the transition of your loved one becomes cause for other actions and emotions. If used properly, psi experiences will aid you in your development; if they are misused, they will get in the way of your yogic development. Misused, they will simply attach you to the material world even more firmly—the world of material possessions and distress. As your psychic abilities become more available, the yamas and niyamas as rules for balanced living in society become even more important. They can be helpful guides for the appropriate utilization of your newfound capacities.

Life as Development and Learning

You can look at your lifetime as a developmental experience. Certainly it is clear in the studies of physical, emotional, and mental development of children that this is so. We have only recently become aware of the developmental stages of adulthood. Books such as D. J. Levinson's *The Seasons of a Man's Life,* R. Gould's *Transformations: Growth and Change in Adult Life,* and others highlight this growing awareness and knowledge. This is very helpful because it enables us to see the entire lifetime as comprised of developmental stages that are still full of promise and creative possibilities. Somatic yoga can be very helpful in making full use of each developmental stage.

One of the most positive ways to face life experiences is in terms of the learning inherent in these experiences. Even with the most bitter experience you can grow, learn, triumph, make the most of it.

When life deals us a blow, we may choose whether we will go down with it or grow with it. I prefer to grow with it. With the learning experiences approach to events, one remains conscious and makes choices so as to minimize the losses and maximize the gains. You can feel the impact of the experience on the development of your inner being or soul.

One of the most helpful concepts I have run into in my reading, thinking, and experiencing is that of "destiny work" or "life's work." I consider your destiny work as a theoretical "best use" of your talents, opportunities, energy. If we could use a computer to analyze all the factors of your personal resources—heredity, environmental opportunities, and so forth—we would be able to plot out the best possible use of those talents, based on an extrapolation of the environmental opportunites that would be offered to you during your lifetime. This is a hypothetical "best fit" because it would never be possible to plot with that kind of accuracy. What we usually do in life, those who have a sense of it, is feel our way along life's path trying to find what seems to be right for us. According to the best fit theory, the closer you get to a life's work that truly fits you, the happier, more effective, and more energetic you will be.

I sometimes like to think of our being in a cosmic feedback system. When we make the right choices, things go well. When we are on the wrong track, things seem to go poorly. It is as if the universe was saying "hot" when we are on the right track and "cold" when we are off the track—like the game of "hot" and "cold" we played as children.

One kind of clue that I use to know I am on the right track is when synchronistic events occur. A synchronistic event is also called a "meaningful coincidence" according to Carl Jung. A meaningful coincidence might be one in which you decide that you want to contact someone, for example, and you pick up the phone and find him on the other end of the phone. He is calling you about the matter that you had in mind and you haven't talked with him in weeks. I would consider that a green light for the project that you had in mind or some variation of it. I try to listen very carefully to what seems to emerge within me as directional leads—hunches, intuitive flashes, fantasies—and then move on them, being very aware of whether the environment seems to support the projects or not—in other words, I use my own common sense to evaluate the situation.

As you do your yoga practice, you will notice the many ways

that it facilitates your development. As psychic abilities become more available to you, this will also enhance your development. You must never forget that the psychic abilities must be used in an ethical and balanced fashion for all concerned. Used in an appropriate manner, the psi experiences of yoga will greatly add to your enjoyment of life and the great journey that it represents.

Conclusion

Somatic Yoga as a Way of Life

Good or bad deeds are not the direct cause of the transformation. They only act as breakers of the obstacles to natural evolution; just as a farmer breaks down the obstacles in a water course, so that water flows through by its own nature.

Patanjali

I entered this class, and my yoga practice, less as a spiritual seeking than as an aid to self-healing and physical fitness. I have found, through my practice and reading, that these go together. I have discovered benefits from my yoga in the forms of lessened anxiety and tension, and increased ability to deal with the things that occur in my everyday life. I'll probably never be a yogi, but, then, I really don't want to be. I'm sure my yoga will continue to help me lead a fuller, happier, and more beneficial life. It makes me feel good!

Yoga student

We have explored yoga psychology from both Western psychology's understanding of Eastern practices and from the research support for the subjective reports that are currently available. We filter our understanding of practices from another culture through our own understandings based on our own experiences and cultural context. This book has attempted to provide the basic principles and practices of somatic yoga with psychophysiological explanations. Development of a unified mind-body state seems to be facilitated by maximum knowledge, of a third-person kind, in conjunction with first-person experiences. When these two kinds of awareness are brought together, there is the beginning of a profound personal transformation.

Yoga practice, no matter what the original goal was, will lead to the transformation of your life context. As you begin to take your development and psychophysiological maintenance into your own hands, there is the thrill of being master of your fate, captain of your ship. There is a great expansion of the sense that you can do practically anything you want to do. And you can. You feel a great increase in your personal power.

This book has attempted to be a smorgasbord of yogic practices. How these practices work physiologically has also been included. You were invited to select practices for your own evolving yoga. The emphasis has been placed on awareness and self-sensing, the bringing together of the first and third person perception for as much time as possible. With practice, you will become increasingly able to maintain that focus. When you are able to do it for any length of time, either in your yoga practice or in your everyday life, you will notice an increase in your effectiveness and available energy. You have been encouraged to feel comfortable with each stage in your yogic development so that you can derive maximum benefit from it.

Our society has been experiencing rapid technological evolution. We cannot continue to evolve at the rate that we have in the past. Our planet does not have limitless resources; our population cannot continue to expand at its accelerating rate. The struggle to "make" it in our society has become less crucial; we have to find ways to relax into our world. Somatic yoga can help you relax and enjoy your life, to really see, hear, taste and savor your experiences rather than substitute quantity of experience for quality.

In modern times, we have become alienated from our environment. We have even become self-conscious about our alienation. Perhaps it will be possible to do something about it. Let's hope so. There is still time. Somatic yoga is an excellent way to begin to get back in touch with nature. It is, in fact, a way of establishing a harmonious rhythm with the forces of nature. As you begin to be more conscious of the air you breathe, for example, you seek more pranic air. As you begin to do your yoga outdoors, you begin to feel the earth and its more organismic sensations. As your senses become more refined and you begin to see and sense your relationship to all of your environment, you begin to appreciate more and more of what the natural world has to offer.

When you confront your mortality, you begin to notice that there is a lifetime to create. Somatic yoga is a powerful means of enabling you to take an active role in the creation of your life.

Some people who study yoga experience its benefits, but drift away from it in time. Others gradually incorporate it into their ways of life. Some individuals find it meaningful to devote their lives to yoga. In India, a person has various stages in his life during which he devotes himself to the dharma of that stage. During his householder stage, he marries, has a family, and participates in the business affairs of the town or village. Later he may leave the ordinary life to seek philosophic and spiritual seclusion.

Some individuals, who feel their lives growing simpler and simpler as they come closer to the yogic way, may choose a life of abstention. Ideally, this is done because the results of yoga become so splendid that it is not a sacrifice, but a going toward what seems to be far more fulfilling. You can make an intellectual decision to live a more ascetic life or you can follow the natural trends inherent in your development.

If your are in the householder period of your life, you are deeply involved with your family, friends, and society. This is a worldly period and must be experienced fully in order to learn from it. During this period, somatic yoga can be an integral part of your life while facilitating your daily activities. At this stage you are a karma yogi or yogini, living a life of service. May you be happy and healthy as you do your work in the world!

Appendix

15 Week Somatic Yoga Program

(See p. 66 for the somatic yoga session format.)

Key to Postures

a	legs up	g	locust
b	half shoulderstand	h	bow
c	sholderstand	i	spinal twist
d	fish	j	yoga mudra
e	plow	k	head-to-knee
f	cobra	l	tree

Week 1   Warmups
          Postures a & b (30 seconds)
          Pranayama—rapid breath
          Pratyahara
          Meditation (5 minutes)

Week 2   Warm-ups
          Postures a, b & c (30 seconds)
          Pranayama
             rapid breath
             same nostril breath 1:4:2 ratio
          Pratyahara
          Meditation (10 minutes)

Week 3   Warm-ups
          Posture a (1 minute)
          Posture b (40 seconds)
          Posture c (1 minute)
          Posture d (30 seconds)

Week 3 (con'd)	Pranayama
	  rapid breath
	  alternate nostril breath 1:4:2 ratio
	Pratyahara
	Meditation (15 minutes)

Week 4	Warm-ups Posture a (1 minute) Posture b (40 seconds) Posture c (1½ minutes) Posture d (1 minute) Posture e (30 seconds) Pranayama (see week 3) Pratyahara Meditation (20 minutes)
Week 5	Warm-ups Posture a (1 minute) Posture b (40 seconds) Posture c (1½ minutes) Posture d (1½ minutes) Posture e (1 minute) Posture f (2 repetitions) Pranayama Pratyahara Meditation (20 minutes)
Week 6	Warm-ups Posture a (1 minute) Posture b (40 seconds) Posture c (2 minutes) Posture d (2 minutes) Posture e (1½ minutes) Posture f (3 repetitions) Posture g (2 repetitions) Pranayama Pratyahara Meditation (20 minutes)

Week 7	Warm-ups Posture a (1 minute) Posture b (40 seconds) Posture c (2½ minutes) Posture d (2½ minute) Posture e (2 minutes) Posture f (3 repetitions) Posture g (3 repetitions) Posture h (2 repetitions) Pranayama Pratyahara Meditation (20 minutes)
Week 8	Warm-ups Posture a (1 minute) Posture b (40 seconds) Posture c (3 minutes) Posture d (3 minute) Posture e (2½ minutes) Posture f (3 repetitions) Posture g (3 repetitions) Posture h (3 repetitions) Posture i (30 seconds each side) Pranayama Pratyahara Meditation (20 minutes)
Week 9	Warm-ups Postures a–d–same as above Posture e (3 minutes) Posture f–h–same as above Posture i (30 seconds each side) Pranayama Pratyahara Meditation (20 minutes)
Week 10	Warm-ups Postures a–i –same as above

Week 10 (con'd)	Posture j (20 seconds) Pranayama Pratyahara Meditation (20 minutes)
Week 11	Warm-ups Postures a–j—same as above Posture k (1 minute) Posture l (20 seconds each side) Pranayama Pratyahara Meditation (20 minutes)
Weeks 12–15	Follow the session format above.

Add additional poses for variety. See books by Vishnudevananda and Swami Satchidananda.

References

Anand, B. K., Chhina, G.S., & Singh, B. Some aspects of electroencephalographic studies in yogis. *EEG and Clinical Neurophysiology,* 1961, 13, 452–456.

Banquet, J. P. Spectral analysis of EEG in meditation. *Electroencephalography and Clinical Neurophysiology,* 1973, 35, 143–151.

Benson, H., Beary, J. F., & Carol, M. P. The relaxation response, *Psychiatry,* 1974, 37, 37–46.

Brown, F. M., Steward, W. S., & Blodgett, J. T. *EEG kappa rhythms during transcendental meditation and possible threshold changes following.* Paper presented to the Kentucky Academy of Science, Richmond, November 13, 1971.

Butter, C. M. *Neuropsychology: The Study of Brain and Behavior.* Monterey, CA: Brooks Cole, 1968.

Carlson, N. *Physiology of Behavior.* Boston: Allyn & Bacon, 1977.

Chaudhuri, H. Yoga psychology. In C. T. Tart (ed.), *Transpersonal Psychologies.* New York: Harper & Row, 1975.

Das, N. N. & Gastant, H. Variations de l'activite electrique du cerveau, du coeur et des muscles squelettiques au cours de la meditation et de l'extase yogique. *EEG,* Supplement, 1955, 6, 211–219.

Dhanaraj, V. H. The effects of yoga and the 5BX fitness plan on selected physiological parameters. (Doctoral dissertation, University of Alberta, 1974).

Feldenkrais, M. *Awareness Through Movement.* New York: Harper & Row, 1972.

Funderburk, J. *Science Studies Yoga: A Review of Physiological Data.* Illinois: Himalayan International Institute of Yoga Science and Philosophy of USA, 1977.

Garoutte, B. Personal Communication, 1988.

Garoutte, B. *Survey of Functional Neuroanatomy.* Greenbrae, CA: Jones Medical Publications, 1987.

Gopal, K. S., Anatharaman, V., Nishith, S. D. & Bhatnagar, O.P. The effect of yogasanas on muscular tone and cardio-respiratory adjustments. *Yoga Life,* 1975, 6(5), 3–11.

Gould, R. *Transformations: Growth and Change in Adult Life.* New York: Simon & Schuster, 1978.

Hanna, T. *The Body of Life.* New York: Alfred Knopf, 1980.

Isherwood, C. *Ramakrishna and His Disciples.* New York: Simon & Schuster, 1970.

Jacobson, E. *Progressive Relaxation* (2nd Ed.). Chicago: University of Chicago Press, 1938.

Jung, C. Synchronicity: An Acausal Connecting Principle (1952). In #8 *The Structure and Dynamics of the Psyche.* In R. F. C. Hull (trans.), *The Collected Works of Carl G. Jung.* Princeton, N.J.: Bollingen Series XX, Princeton University Press, 1960.

Kasamatsu, A. & Hirai, R. An electroencephalographic study on the zen meditation (zazen). In C. T. Tart (ed.), *Altered States of Consciousness.* Garden City, New York: Doubleday, 1975.

Kuvalayananda, Swami & Vinekar, S. L. *Yogic Therapy: Its Basic Principles and Methods.* New Delhi: Ministry of Health, Government of India, 1971.

LeShan, L. *The Medium, the Mystic and the Physicist: Toward a General Theory of the Paranormal.* New York: Viking, 1973.

LeShan, L. *Toward a General Theory of the Paranormal.* New York: Parapsychological Monographs, Parapsychology Foundation, 1969.

Levinson, D. J. *The Seasons of a Man's Life.* New York: Knopf, 1978.

Ludwig, A. M. Altered States of Consciousness. In C. T. Tart (ed.), *Altered States of Consciousness.* Garden City, New York: Doubleday, 1975.

MacLean. P. D. *A Triune Concept of the Brain and Behaviour.* Papers presented at Queen's University, Kingston, Ontario. February 1969 by V. A. Kral and others. Published for Ontario Mental Health Foundation by University of Toronto Press, 1973.

Mishra, R. S. *Fundamentals of Yoga: A Handbook of Theory, Practice, Application.* New York: The Julian Press, 1959.

Mishra, R. S. *Yoga Sutras: The Textbook of Yoga Psychology.* Garden City, New York: Anchor Press/Doubleday, 1973.

Monroe, R. *Journeys Out of the Body.* New York: Doubleday, 1971.

Moses, R. Effect of yoga on flexibility and respiratory measures of vital capacity and breath holding time. (Doctoral dissertation, University of Oregon, 1972).

Patel, C. 12-month follow-up of yoga and bio-feedback in the management of hypertension. *Lancet,* 1975, *1,* 62–64.

Patel, C. Yoga and bio-feedback in the management of hypertension. *Lancet*, 1973, 2, 1053–1055.

Patel, C. & North, W. R. S. Randomised controlled trial of yoga and bio-feedback in the management of hypertension. *Lancet*, 1975, 2, 93–95.

Prabhavananda, Swami & Isherwood, C. *How to Know God: The Yoga of Patanjali*. New York: Signet Books, 1953.

Ram Das. *Be Here Now*. San Cristobal, New Mexico: Lama Foundation, 1971.

Rhine, J. B. *Extra-Sensory Perception*. Boston: Humphries, 1934.

Satchidananda, Yogiraj Sri Swami. *Integral Yoga Hatha*. New York: Holt, Rinehart & Winston, 1970.

Schmeidler, G. The psychic personality. In E. D. Mitchell (ed.), *Psychic Exploration: A Challenge for Science*. New York: G. P. Putnam's Sons, 1974.

Schwartz, G. E. *Pros and cons of meditation*. Paper presented at the American Psychological Association Convention, Montreal, August 1973.

Stanford, R. G. *The integration of cognitive processing factors: ESP in life situations*. Paper presented at the AAAS Annual Meeting, Washington, D.C., December, 1972 as part of the symposium, Understanding Parapsychological Phenomena: A Survey of Four Possible Areas of Integration, sponsored by the Parapsychological Association.

Tart, C. T. (ed.) *Transpersonal Psychologies*. New York: Harper & Row, 1975.

Underhill, E. *Mysticism* (12th Edition). New York: E. P. Dutton, 1961.

Vishnudevananda, Swami. *The Complete Illustrated Book of Yoga*. New York: Crown Publishing Co., 1988.

Wood, E. *Yoga*. Harmondsworth, Middlesex, England: Penguin Books, 1962.

Wood, E. *Yoga Wisdom* (*Yoga Dictionary*). New York: Philosophical Library, 1970.

ABOUT THE AUTHOR

Eleanor Criswell, EdD, has been a student of yoga psychology and meditation for 27 years. She has taught yoga psychology in the Psychology Department of Sonoma State University for 20 years. She has published articles on yoga psychology in magazines and journals during that time. As managing editor of *Somatics*, a magazine-journal of the bodily arts and sciences, she has a strong interest in furthering the awareness of the possibilities for health and well-being inherent in mind-body integration. To that end she has also trained teachers of yoga psychology.